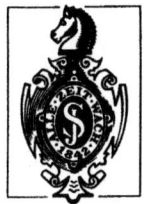

Georg Kamm   Toni Graf-Baumann

Machame
Anaesthesia Notebook
for Medical Auxiliaries

**With Special Emphasis
on the Developing Countries**

With 89 Figures and 14 Tables

Springer-Verlag
Berlin Heidelberg GmbH 1982

Georg Kamm
Head of Dept. of Anaesthesia
Machame Hospital, Box 3044
Moshi, Tanzania

Toni Graf-Baumann
SIFKU-Institut, Holtenauerstraße
D-2300 Kiel

CIP-Kurztitelaufnahme der Deutschen Bibliothek
Kamm, Georg:
Machame anaesthesia notebook for medical auxiliaries: with special emphasis
on the developing countries / Georg Kamm; Toni Graf-Baumann. – Berlin;
Heidelberg; New York: Springer, 1982.
ISBN 978-3-540-09055-7   ISBN 978-3-642-67101-2 (eBook)
DOI 10.1007/978-3-642-67101-2

NE: Graf-Baumann, Toni

Printing and binding: K. Triltsch, Würzburg
2127/3140-543210

To Professor Dr. Rudolf Frey

and to all Tanzanians who joined with me in striving for the one and main purpose in performing anaesthesia under the motto:

Divinum est sedare dolorem

It is divine to abolish pain

Foreword

The advances in the field of anaesthesiology and reanimation have contributed in all developed countries to the decrease in deaths occurring on the operating table (exitus in tabula), from the ratio 1:100 (in the nineteenth century) down to approximately 1:1000 (in the first half of the twentieth century) and finally to approximately 1: 10 000 (nowadays).

Numerous human lives were saved not only through the introduction of new medicine and methods but even more so by better training for the doctors and nurses who apply these new techniques.

I am happy about the splendid initiative of my student and friend Georg Kamm, which has now made these advances accessible to the developing countries. He knows very well how to make his colleagues understand the theory and the practical side of modern anaesthesiology, under the most difficult conditions and in a completely different world, to such an extent that today in his country all of his patients are given the benefit of the advances of medicine.

There is nothing more rewarding for an academic teacher than to see how his students continue developing his ideas and spread them far and wide. I am therefore happy and proud to write this foreword for Georg Kamm, one of the pioneers of anaesthesiology in Africa.

R. Frey

Preface

The intention of this book is to give the necessary knowledge for medical auxiliaries performing anaesthesia, with special emphasis on developing countries. I do not want to provide another textbook on anaesthesia; this should be a work manual. I have only included the information which from my experience is absolutely necessary *for any medical auxiliary* to assist with, or in performing, anaesthesia.

It is my hope that this booklet will bring understanding of the drugs and agents used, and will help in the training and in the performance of different techniques, with the aim of achieving practical, simple and safe anaesthesia.

G. Kamm

Acknowledgements

Through the continuous support and encouragement of my esteemed teacher and friend Prof. Rudolf Frey F.F.A.R.C.S., I have been in the position to start and successfully finish this handbook on anaesthesia. It is in my sincere gratitude that it is dedicated to him with thanks. To all my other teachers who helped to build up my knowledge and my personality I also extend my sincere thanks.

I am indebted to many of my colleagues and friends. My little booklet has greatly profited from the experience and masterful corrections of Mr. Peter Bewes of the K.C.M.C., Moshi, who provided much constructive critisism. I want to thank Peter Timmermanns, Ruediger Kilian, F. Finsterer and M. Scudder for giving their expert advice and many practical comments.

I would also like to acknowledge here the 12 years of collaboration with my colleague Dr. Rudolf Schmidt of Machame Hospital, who from the very beginning of my career as an anaesthetist at this hospital never failed to help me with indispensable advice and valuable contributions to attain today's success, as well as my friends Mr. J. Urasa and E. Msuya.

I wish to thank Mrs. Renata Kuehne from Jena, DDR, for her skill and patience in transferring the jungle of my papers into plain and acceptable language and for typing it all on stencils. Many thanks also to Mrs. Lilian for copying the many stencils that make up this book.

Finally my heartiest thanks to Maria, my dear wife, for helping me in ever so many ways.

G. Kamm

Table of Contents

Illustration Credit

The following figures have been redrawn from originals in "Gorgaß·Ahnefeld, Der Rettungssanitäter", Springer-Verlag 1980; Figs. 14.2–14.6, 14.8.

Chapter 1

A Short Review of the Anatomy and Physiology of the Respiratory System

A knowledge of the respiratory system and its physiology is important to the anaesthetist because a large number of drugs used in anaesthesia interfere with the normal physiological function of the respiratory and circulatory systems. The anaesthetist is therefore responsible for the adequate maintenance of these systems and some knowledge of anatomy and physiology is essential.

1.1 Anatomy (see Fig. 1.1)

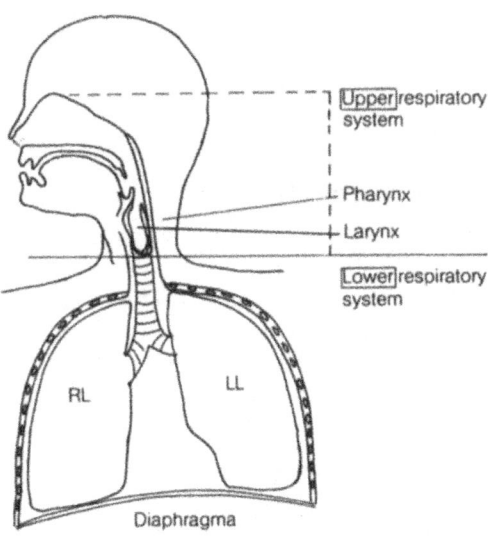

Upper respiratory system

Pharynx

Larynx

Lower respiratory system

RL

LL

Diaphragma

Fig. 1.1. The respiratory system

1

1.2 Physiology

1.2.1 Upper Respiratory System

The nose and pharynx are responsible for warming up, humidifying and purifying the inspired air. This is to be considered during anaesthesia, as in an unconscious patient an airway or an endotracheal tube prevents these normal functions. The possibility of contaminating the air reaching the lungs with dust or bacteria is therefore increased. As shown in Fig. 1.2, in an anaesthetised patient, lying down, the soft tissues tend to fall back and may block the upper respiratory tract (see also Chap. 4).

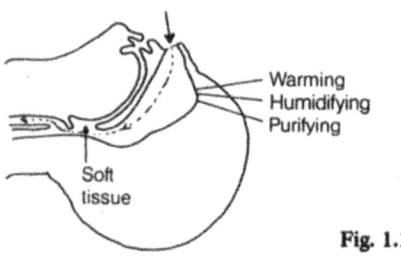

Warming
Humidifying
Purifying

Soft
tissue

Fig. 1.2

1.2.2 Lower Respiratory System

1.2.2.1 Larynx

The larynx is an important organ for the anaesthetist as it is the entrance to the trachea. The larynx consists of the epiglottis, the vocal cords, the aryepiglottis and the glottis (see Fig. 1.3). The arytenoid cartilages are responsible for the function of the larynx. During normal breathing the cords move apart and during swallowing the glottis reflexively closes the airway.

Spasms of the larynx are caused by:
a) Irritant vapours, e.g. ether
b) Foreign material, e.g. tracheal tube
c) Vagal stimulus

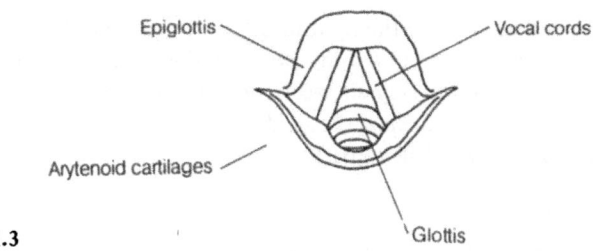

Fig. 1.3

1.2.2.2 Trachea

In an average adult the trachea is 10-12 cm long and supported by U-shaped cartilagenous arches. The epithelium is a ciliated mucosa and is responsible for removing upwards the secretions of the trachea and lungs.

1.2.2.3 Bronchi

The right bronchus is almost a direct continuation of the trachea, while the left one diverges more sharply (see Fig. 1.4). Therefore an endotracheal tube, if placed too deep, tends to enter the right bronchus and in consequence does not provide adequate ventilation for both lungs (see Chap. 4). The bronchi are surrounded by smooth muscle tissue and spasm of this tissue results in bronchial spasm or in bronchial asthma. These can be caused by histamine liberation, vagal stimuli, etc.

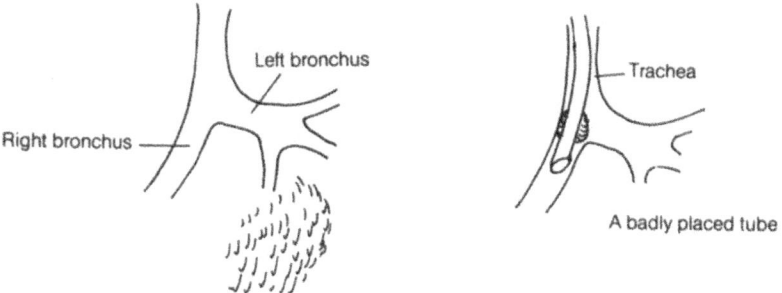

Fig. 1.4

1.2.2.4 Lungs

The function of the lungs is both the exchange of gases (carbon dioxide and oxygen) between air and the blood capillaries, and the maintenance of pH. The exchange therefore takes place across the alveolar membrane. Each lung is

3

divided into lobes: the right lung has three, the left lung has two lobes. The lungs are enclosed in a shiny skin called pleura pulmonalis. The lungs contain 300–750 million tiny air sacs called alveoli, which are closely surrounded by blood capillaries. (Spread out, the surface of the capillaries would cover the area of a basket-ball court.)

1.2.3 Mechanism of Ventilation

By the active enlargement of the thorax (contraction of the intercostal muscles) and the descent of the diaphragm, air is sucked into the lungs. This is the inspiratory phase (see Fig. 1.5). As soon as the inspiratory muscles relax, the ribs fall back and the arch of the diaphragm rises: the thoracic cavity becomes smaller and the lungs fall back. This is the expiratory phase (see Fig. 1.6).

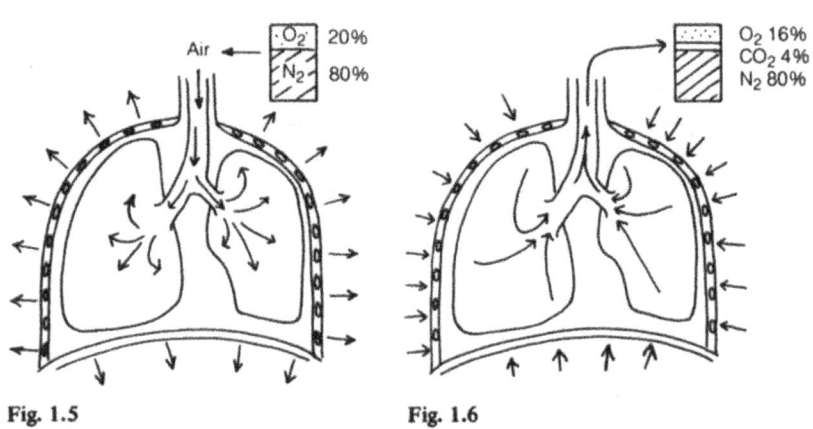

Fig. 1.5   Fig. 1.6

1.2.4 Regulation of Respiration

Respiration is mainly controlled by the central respiratory centre in the medulla, which is influenced by:

    a) O_2-lack or excess
    b) CO_2-lack or excess
    c) Change of blood pH
    d) Chemoreceptor (O_2 and CO_2 concentration)
    e) Pressure receptors (blood pressure stimuli)

f) Stretch receptors (alveoli)

g) Sensory stimuli from the whole (pain and temperature)

h) Brain reflexes

The increase in CO_2 sensitises the respiratory centre and the increase in O_2 reduces the activity of the respiratory centres.

1.2.5 Normal Respiratory Rate

Newborn: 40 breaths/min

Children: 20 breaths/min

Adults: 12-16 breaths/min

The ventilation capacity can be divided into:

a) Tidal volume — the amount of air passing in and out for each normal breath (10 ml/kg body wt.)

b) Vital capacity — the maximum inspiratory and expiratory volume

c) Residual volume — the air always remaining in the lungs

d) The minute volume — the volume of air passing in and out per min (average 1 litre/kg body wt.)

e) Respiratory rate — the frequency of respiration per min

(see Fig. 1.7)

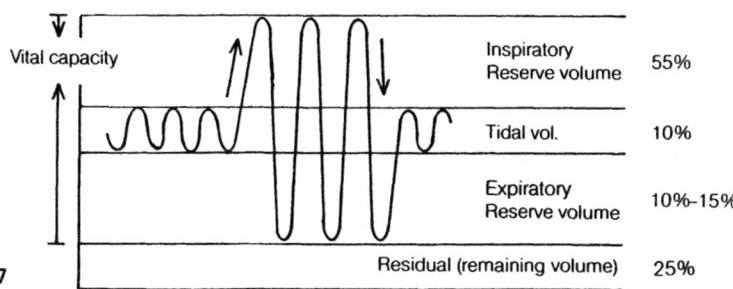

Fig. 1.7

For example an average adult of 60 kg will have a tidal volume of 10 x 60 = 600 ml. So the minute volume will be 600 x 12 = 7.2 litre/min. The minute volume can also be found from the normogram (after Redfort). The function of the lungs is to maintain with all their ability, the normal tension of O_2 and CO_2 and normal pH in the arterial and venous blood.

Arterial: pO_2 =   100 mmHg

        pCO_2 =   40 mmHg

Venous: pO_2 =   40 mmHg

        pCO_2 =   46 mmHg

5

The ability of the lungs to maintain the normal tension of gases in the blood depends upon:

a) Ventilation — the amount and concentration of O_2 and CO_2 reaching the alveoli

b) Diffusion — the ability of the gases to exchange between the alveoli and the capillaries

c) Perfusion — the amount of pulmonary blood and haemoglobin passing through the capillaries (see Fig. 1.8)

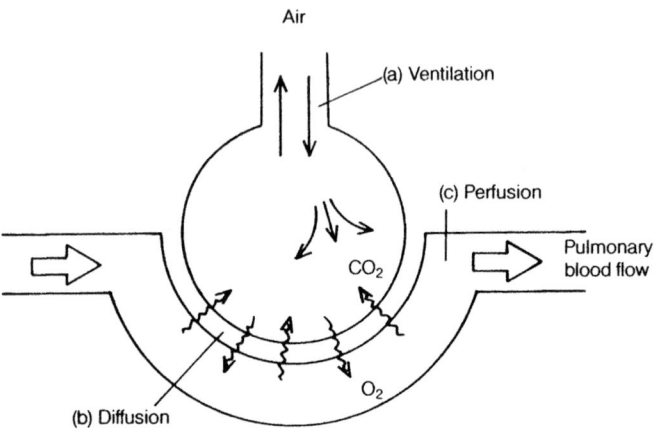

Fig. 1.8

1.2.5.1 Ventilation

The important factor is the amount, in particular, of oxygen reaching the alveoli. Not all the tidal air reaches the alveoli. Tidal air can be divided into alveolar air (2.5 litre/min/m^2 body surface) and dead space (body weight in kg — 2 ml). The dead space consists of the mouth, nose, pharynx, trachea, bronchi and, during anaesthesia with anaesthetic equipment, the dead space of the equipment (see Fig. 1.9).

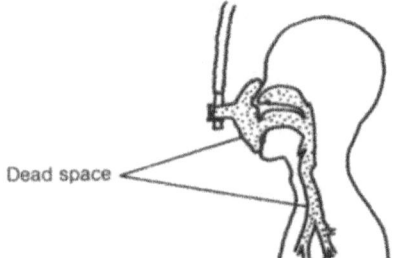

Dead space

Fig. 1.9

In anaesthesia alveolar ventilation = 600 ml tidal volume – 150 ml ds – 50 ml ds from anaesthesia machine = 400 ml (about 60% of the tidal volume). In anaesthesia tidal volume = 600 ml; dead space (ds) = 150 ml. Therefore, alveolar ventilation = 600 –150 = 450 ml.

In shallow respiration where the volume goes down from 600 to 300 or even 130 ml, but frequency is going up, the alveolar ventilation consequently goes down drastically. For example:

300 Tidal volume x frequency 20 per min = 6000; 200 ds x frequency 20 per min = 4000.
6000 –4000 = 2000 ml/min, which is not enough!

In the case of hyperventilation (increased respiratory frequency and therefore reduced tidal volume) the proportion of dead space increases. This is an important factor to be considered in anaesthesia with spontaneous respiration (see Fig. 1.10).

1.2.5.2 Diffusion

Gas exchange is a positive process. The diffusing gases have to pass through the alveolar epithelium, the interstitial fluid and the capillary endothelium.

Pathological conditions of one or more of these three layers will impair diffusion. The alveolar epithelium may be thickened or covered by fluid or pus, for instance from a lung disease. The interstitial fluid and the capillary endothelium may become less permeable due to heart failure or disease, etc.

1.2.5.3 Perfusion

Of final importance is the flow rate and carrying capacity of the blood for carrying away oxygen and returning carbon dioxide (pulmonary bloodflow). The flow rate can be reduced by heart disease or failure or by congenital heart conditions. If the blood flow is too slow the oxygen is not carried quickly enough to the body cells. On the other hand if the carrying capacity is not large enough (haemoglobin), not enough oxygen will be carried to the body cells (e.g. anaemia). The ideal relationship between ventilation and perfusion is:

Alveolar ventilation = 4 litre/min
Pulmonary blood flow = 5 litre/min

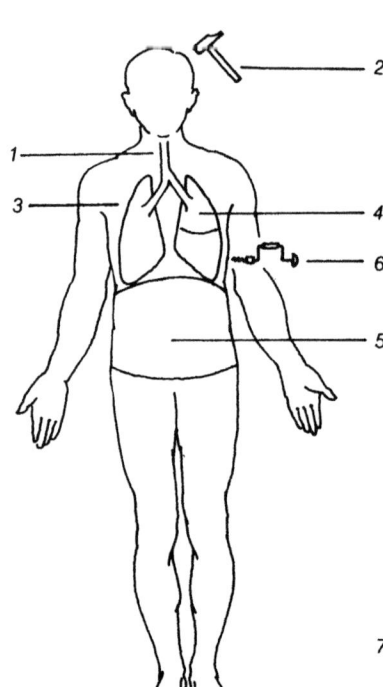

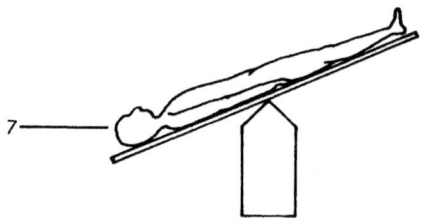

Fig. 1.10. Cases of reduced ventilation (hypoventilation): *1* obstruction anywhere in the respiratory tract (see Chap. 6), *2* drugs which depress the respiratory centres, e.g. morphine, *3* respiratory muscle weakness, e.g. under muscle relaxant, *4* pathology of lung or chest, e.g. pneumonia or crushed chest, *5* abdominal swelling O.B., *6* pain in chest or abdomen, *7* position of patient during anaesthesia

1.3 Oxygen

The most important substance in the air is oxygen. The oxygen proportions and tensions are:

Inspired air 20%	158 mmHg
Expired air 16%	116 mmHg
Alveolar air 15%	103 mmHg
Arterial blood	100 mmHg
Venous blood	40 mmHg

The normal consumption of O_2 is 4-6 ml/kg/min in adults and 7 ml/kg /min in children. 1 g haemoglobin is able to carry 1.34 ml O_2. *Oxygen deficiency in the body weakens and finally stops all functions.* Initially the body tries to compensate for the deficiency by hyperventilation (dilatation of the coronary vessels), raising the pulse rate and increasing the blood flow to the brain, but if the deficiency worsens, conditions deteriorate and the body function ceases. Damage caused to the central nervous system by O_2 deficiency is irreversible. Possible causes of insufficient O_2 in inspired air:

a) Insufficient O_2 in inspired air
b) Respiratory obstruction
c) Inadequate ventilation
d) Lung disease
e) Perfusion failure
f) Anaemia

Remember: during anaesthesia, oxygen concentration has to be kept high.

1.4 Anatomy and Physiology of the Autonomic Nerve System

Since many drugs used in anaesthesia have a strong action on the autonomic nerve system, a short revision of the physiology of the autonomic nerve system is shown in Fig. 1.11.

Parasympathetic nerve system   Sympathetic nerve system

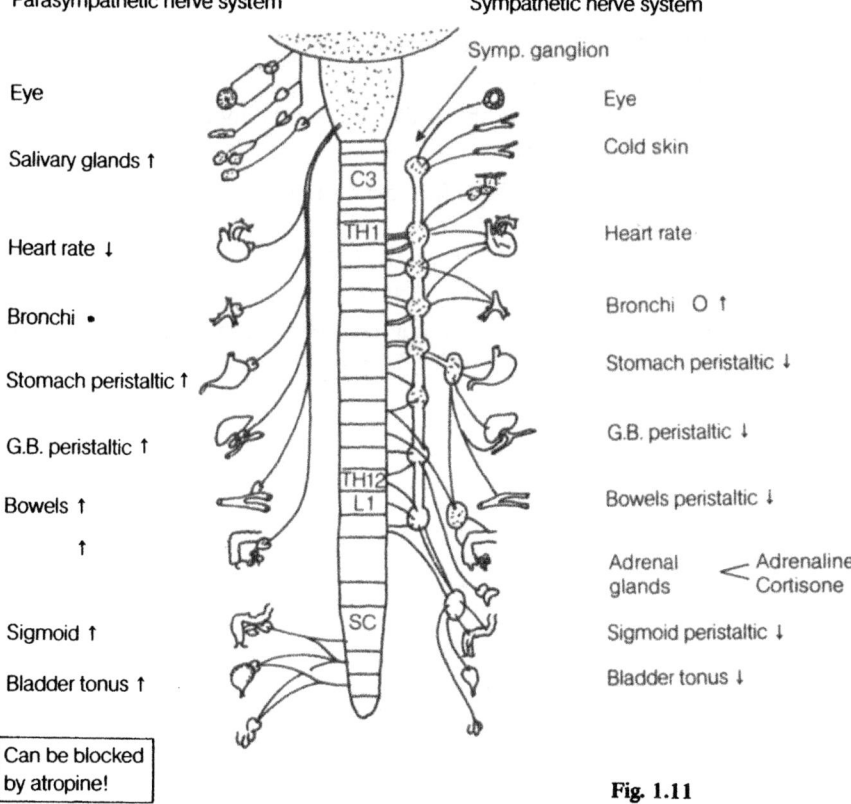

Symp. ganglion

Eye

Salivary glands ↑

Heart rate ↓

Bronchi •

Stomach peristaltic ↑

G.B. peristaltic ↑

Bowels ↑

↑

Sigmoid ↑

Bladder tonus ↑

Can be blocked
by atropine!

Eye

Cold skin

Heart rate

Bronchi O ↑

Stomach peristaltic ↓

G.B. peristaltic ↓

Bowels peristaltic ↓

Adrenal glands ⟨ Adrenaline / Cortisone

Sigmoid peristaltic ↓

Bladder tonus ↓

Fig. 1.11

9

Chapter 2

Pharmacology of General Anaesthesia

Compounds of many different chemical types can induce general anaesthesia. Anaesthesia is a reversible state of paralysation of cells in the central nervous system (CNS) causing unconsciousness, analgesia and reduction of reflexes. The reversible state of paralysation of the CNS by general anaesthetic drugs has been described by Goodman and Gillman as an "anatomical regular descending paralysis" of the cortex, basal ganglia, cerebellum and spinal cord. The effect of an anaesthesia drug depends on the concentration of cells; the concentration, however, depends on:

a) Absorption   c) Demobilisation
b) Distribution   d) Excretion

The removal of anaesthetic agents depends on the following types of chemical breakdown and fate:

a) Hydrolysis (fixation of H_2O (chemical addition of H_2O)
b) Fixation
c) Demethylation (chemical removal of CH_3)
d) Oxidation (chemical addition of oxygen)

There are different stages of anaesthesia, according to the paralysation of cells in the CNS classified by Guedel as follows (Table 2.1):

a) Reflexes
b) Respiration
c) Muscle tonus

Table 2.1

	Pupils	Respiration		Muscle tonus	Remarks
		costal	dia-phrag.		
Stage I	◉				Amnesia
Stage II	⬤				Excitement
Stage III₁	◉				Surg. Anaesth.
Stage III₂	◉				
Stage III₃	⬤				
Stage III₄	⬤				

Anaesthesia can be achieved by: (Table 2.1)

A) Local anaesthesia, which means blocking the sensoric impulses from
   a localised area, causing:

   a) Analgesia (no pain)
   b) Muscle relaxation

B) General anaesthesia, which means:

   a) Amnesia (not aware)
   b) Analgesia (no pain)
   c) Muscle relaxation

To these ends, the methods used to achieve general anaesthesia are:

   a) Inhalation
   b) Intravenous anaesthesia (IV)
   c) Combined anaesthesia, using (a) + (b) and an addition of
   d) Muscle relaxant

2.1 Inhalation Anaesthesia

Inhalation narcotics are agents which are inhaled into the alveoli, to diffuse
into the blood from where they will be transported to the cells in the CNS.
They are mainly eliminated through exhalation rather than by metabolism in
the body. The anaesthetic depth depends upon the saturation in the brain. For
induction high concentrations are needed, because the anaesthetic diffuses in
the whole body. If sufficient saturation has been reached, lower concentrations
are adequate to maintain anaesthesia (see Table 2.1).

2.1.1 Ether

Ether ($C_2H_5 - 0 - C_2H_5$) is a synthetic of catalytic action of sulphuric acid
+ ethyl alcohol: a colourless volatile liquid with a pungent smell. It boils at
36.6^oC and is highly inflammable. With our many new anaesthetic drugs, methods and agents, the words of John Snow about ether in 1858 are still valid:
"I hold it therefore to be most impossible that death from this agent can occur
in the hand of a medical man who is applying it with ordinary intelligence and
attention". Ether is cheap, an excellent analgesic muscle relaxant with a wide
narcotic range. Its only disadvantage is a long induction and recovery period.

2.1.1.1 Effects on the Central Respiratory System (CRS)

Ether is not a respiratory depressant. In the surgical stage of anaesthesia, the sensitivity of the respiratory centre to changes in CO_2 tension rises. The respiratory frequence increases, which may result from the irritating effect of ether on the mucous membranes. Ether is a strong irritant on the respiratory tract mucosa, resulting in hypersecretion: saliva production and cough. This can be observed if ether anaesthesia is being induced too quickly. Premedication with atropine is therefore essential. Ether, however, has a bronchodilatating effect. *Induction of anaesthesia with ether is difficult and unpleasant.*

2.1.1.2 Effect on the Cardio-Vascular System (CVS)

Ether has very little or no effect on the myocardium; therefore it is not contraindicated for patients with myocardial disease. Only in deep ether anaesthesia is there a fall of blood pressure (B P) due to the relaxation of the vascular muscle tonus. Arrythmia under ether anaesthesia may occur, but is rare.

2.1.1.3 Muscle Relaxation

Ether *reduces* the tone in the voluntary muscle tissues and the uterus. Since ether has a curarine-like effect the dosage of muscle relaxant under ether anaesthesia has to be reduced. Ether is a parasympathetic depressant while at the same time a sympathetic stimulant, resulting in increase of noradrenaline, causing:

a) Increase of pulse rate
b) Increase of glycogen, which means rise of blood sugar
c) Increase of coronary arterial dilatation
d) Increase of respiratory rate
e) Dilatation of the gut and inhibitions of its movement

Often ether anaesthesia is followed by nausea and vomiting, which can be eliminated by low concentration and proper premedication.

2.1.1.4 Disadvantages of Ether

a) Slow and unpleasant induction period
b) Severe saliva production
c) Prolonged recovery period with frequent post-operative vomiting
d) Inflammable, even explosive if mixed with O_2 and N_2O.

2.1.1.5 Advantages of Ether

a) Low toxicity with a wide therapeutic range
b) Not a cardiac or respiratory depressant
c) Good muscle relaxation
d) Cheap and available everywhere

2.1.1.6 Dosage of Ether

Concentration of 8%-10% for a period of up to 20 min is needed to reach the surgical stage of anaesthesia. For maintenance, an ether concentration of 4%-8% is sufficient.
Ether is mainly excreted unchanged by the lungs.

2.1.2 Halothane

Halothane is a clear, sweet-smelling fluid (2 Brom − 2 chlor 1.1.1. Trifluoraethan). Its specific gravity is 1.86 and it boils at $50.2^{o}C$; it is non-inflammable and contains 0.01% thymol for stabilisation. *Halothane is a quick-acting anaesthetic agent with a short induction and recovery period.* The stage of central depression is four times stronger than in ether and the range of therapeutic dosage is therefore much smaller. Halothane is a hypnotic with a poor analgesic and muscle relaxing effect.

2.1.2.1 Effect on the CRS

Halothane is a powerful respiratory depressant. It produces a progressive decrease of the respiratory minute volume which will result in an increase of CO_2 concentration in the blood under halothane anaesthesia. The respiratory centre becomes irresponsive to its stimulation. Halothane has no irritating effect on the respiratory tract mucosa and no increase of saliva production. Since it is not inflammable it is widely used in chest surgery and in patients with chest diseases, in combination with muscle relaxants as well as induction agent.

2.1.2.2 Effect on the CVS

Halothane depresses the myocardium. The concentrations of halothane necessary to maintain the surgical stage of anaesthesia without a muscle relaxant reduce the cardial output, together with a fall of arterial B P and elevation of venous pressure. Halothane sensitises the heart, like chloroform, against adrenaline causing arrhythmia. Be careful with patients in stress. Do not use it after adrenaline infiltration. Halothane stimulates the vagus, resulting in

13

bradycardia (premedication atropine). If the halothane concentration is kept low, e.g. not more than 0.8% volume, none of the negative effects are very predominant. There has been much talk of the toxic effect of halothane on the liver but so far there is no definite proof that halothane causes liver damage. Investigations are, however, going on.

2.1.2.3 Excretion and Fate

The drug is excreted mainly unchanged by the lungs in the expiratory air.

2.1.2.4 Disadvantages of Halothane

    a) High cost
    b) Strong respiratory and cardiac depressant with a small therapeutic range
    c) Bradycardia and arrhythmia
    d) Hypotensive effect
    e) Cannot be used after failure of local anaesthesia with adrenaline

2.1.2.5 Advantages of Halothane

    a) Short induction and recovery period
    b) No irritation of the respiratory tract mucosa
    c) Can be used on diabetic patients
    d) Not inflammable

2.1.2.6 Clinical Use

Considering its pharmacological properties, halothane is a suitable agent in combination anaesthesia with muscle relaxants, where it is especially used as a hypnotic. It is also suitable as an induction agent in children. Since halothane counteracts many of the disadvantages of ether, it can be used together with ether for induction (see Chap. 4).

2.1.2.7 Dosage

Concentration of 2%-3% over a period of 5-10 min to produce the surgical stage of anaesthesia. For maintenance 1%-1.5% (see Summary Fig. 2.2).

2.1.3 Trilene

Trilene is a colourless liquid (trichloro-ethylene = $HClC - CCl_2$) smelling like chloroform; not inflammable, but cannot be used with soda lime closed circle (very toxic). Trilene is a good analgesic with a poor hypnotic effect. With normal therapeutic dosage it is difficult to reach the surgical stage of anaesthesia. Arrhythmia occurs under Trilene anaesthesia, especially in the case of high CO_2 and in combination with adrenaline. Otherwise Trilene has very little effect on the cardiovascular system. Respiration becomes rapid and *shallow*. Especially under spontaneous respiration there is danger of dead space ventilation with a rapid increase of CO_2. Never use *Trilene with soda lime*.

2.1.4 Gas

Nitrous oxide (N_2O) is a colourless, slightly sweet-smelling gas, obtainable in blue gas cylinders (except in the United States and Germany). It is 1.5 times heavier than air, which brings the danger of re-anaesthetation after anaesthesia. As long as N_2O is applied with sufficient O_2 (at least 25%), it has no significant effect on any system. N_2O is mainly used in combination with anaesthesia (O_2 + N_2O + halothane + muscle relaxant). Nitrous oxide is non-inflammable. It is a good analgesic, a weak hypnotic and a poor relaxant.

2.1.4.1 Use

   a) A substitute in combination anaesthesia
   b) An analgesic to relieve pain (50% O_2 + 50% N_2O)
   c) An analgesic for dental extraction

Table 2.2. Summary

Expense		Resp.	Car.v.	Anal.	Hypn.	Muscle r.	Ind./Rec.		Infl.	Use
cheap	Ether	$\emptyset$	$\emptyset$	+	+	++	sl.	sl.	yes	G.A.
expens.	Halothan	↓	↓	$\emptyset$	++	$\emptyset$	quick		no	Ind.+G.A.
expens.	N_2O	$\emptyset$	$\emptyset$	++	+	$\emptyset$	quick		no	Ind.+G.A.
cheap	Trilene	↓	$\emptyset$	+	+	$\emptyset$	quick		no	Ind.+G.A.

2.2 Intravenous Anaesthesia

2.2.1 Barbiturates

Barbiturates are chemically found when urea reacts with malonic acid (see Fig. 2.1). Barbiturates can be divided into four groups (see Table 2.3). The shor-

Urea   Malonic acid   **Fig. 2.1**

ter the action the greater the amount destroyed in the liver. In anaesthesia the ultra- and short-acting barbiturates are of major interest because of their quick action and short duration. They are, therefore, easier to control.

Table 2.3

Group	Barbiturate	Time of onset	Duration	Dosage	Remarks
I. *Long acting*	Phenobarbital (Luminal)	30 min	6-8 hours	1-3 mg/kg	Long act. sedat
II. *Intermediate action*	Amobarbital	not in use	–	–	–
III. *Short action*	Pentobarbitone Pentobarbital	1-3 min	4 hours	2-3 mg/kg	Induction of sleep
IV. *Ultra-short action*	Thiopentone Thiopental	30 s	2 hours (30 min)	4 mg/kg	of anaesthesia

2.2.1.1 The Effect on the CNS

The drug reaches the brain within 30 s, except in old age and where the circulation is slower, *producing hypnosis (sleep) without analgesis*. The drug is quickly distributed in the body, resulting in a fall of the concentration of the drug in the cells of the CNS so that consciousness returns but the drug is slowly eliminated.

Barbiturates are hypnotica with no analgetic or muscle relaxing effect. If there is analgesis or muscle relaxation in barbiturate-mono-anaésthesia, it is a result of severe depression of the CNS associated with depression of the CRS and the CVS (Table 2.4).

Table 2.4 Summary. Anaesthetic drugs

Drug	Hypnosis	Analgesia	Relaxation	R.S.	C.V.S.	Dosage	Duration
Barbiturate (Thiopentone)	+++	$\emptyset$	$\emptyset$	↓	↓	3-4 mg/kg B W	5-20 min
Ketalar	++	++	–	–	↑	2 mg/kg B W	10 min
Propanidid	+++	(+)	(+)	–	–	7 mg/kg B W	3-4 min

2.2.1.2 Effects on the CRS

Barbiturates are CRS depressants. Every barbiturate anaesthesia or induction produces a respiratory depression (see Fig. 2.2) and therefore interferes dras-

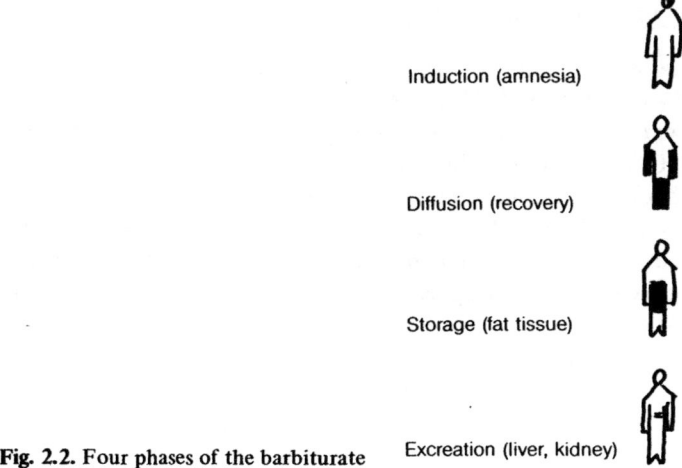

Induction (amnesia)

Diffusion (recovery)

Storage (fat tissue)

Fig. 2.2. Four phases of the barbiturate   Excreation (liver, kidney)

tically with the normal function of the respiratory system. Barbiturates depress the CRS and therefore the centre is irresponsible to the specific stimulation of CO_2 increase. Reduction of R.M.V. (Respiratory Minute Volume) by barbiturate anaesthetica is associated with

a) Increase of CO_2 with no response of the CNS

b) Decrease of O_2
c) Respiratory acidity with fall of pH to 7.3; this can lead to severe complications even after anaesthesia (Fig. 2.3)

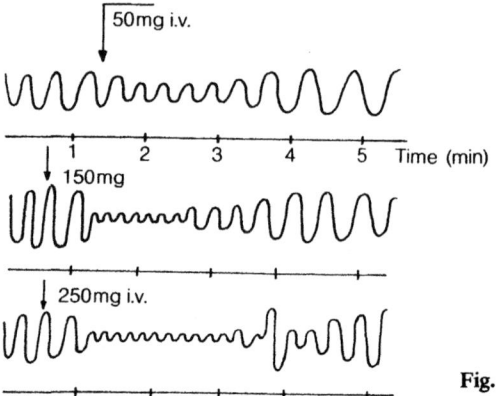

Fig. 2.3

2.2.1.3 Effects on the CVS

Barbituration directly depreses the myocardium, which results in a reduction of the cardial output. This is associated with depression of the central vasotonic centres, which causes a fall of BP even after a small dosage of barbiturate (30% -50%) (see Fig. 2.4). In a hypotonic and older patient, this can easily lead to shock and complications of the CVS. It is, however, reported that barbiturates do not cause arrythmia. Barbiturates, especially by IV application, stimulate the vagus nerve, which explains the tendency for bradycardia and laryngo-broncho spasms (atropine). Induction of barbiturate anaesthesia on asthma patients is therefore contraindicated. Barbiturates cross the placenta immediately. Dosages of not more than 3 mg/kg body wt. have no significant effect on the infant. It also depends on the time between the application and the delivery of the child. The longer the time, the more of the drug will go back to the mother's circulation and will be metabolised (see Chap. 9).

2.2.1.4 Metabolism

10%-20% of Pentothal is metabolised in the liver and 80%-90% is excreted by the kidneys as urea, which will increase the blood urea nitrogen.

2.2.1.5 Advantages of Barbiturates

a) Quick introduction

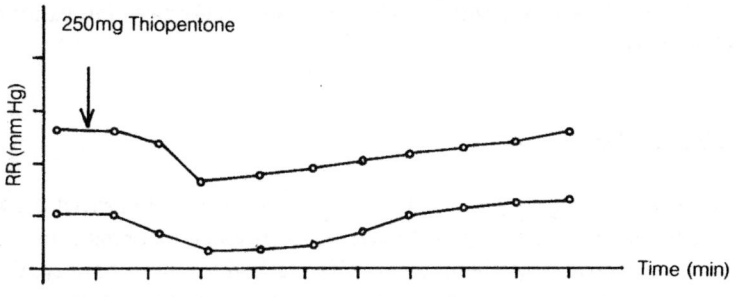

Fig. 2.4

b) Comfortable for the patient
c) Relatively cheap

2.2.1.6 Disadvantages of Barbiturates (see Fig. 2.5)

a) Respiratory and cardio depressant
b) Larynx and bronchospasms
c) Difficulty in determining proper dosage
d) With promethazine and morphine the toxic effect of barbiturate is enhanced.

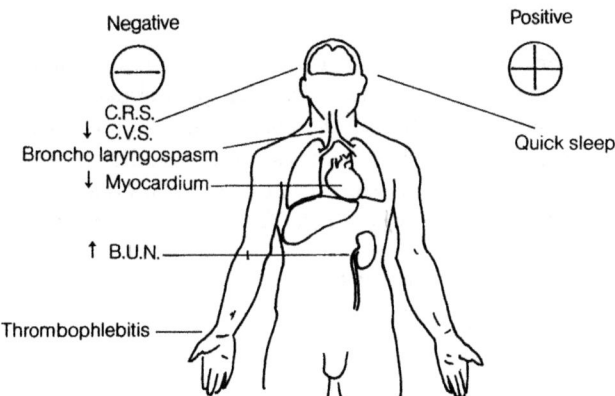

Fig. 2.5

2.2.1.7 Contraindications

a) Severe liver diseases
b) High blood urea
c) Shock and hypotonia
d) Heart failure where the cardial output is already restricted
e) Where there is no possibility of artificial respiration

Sir R. Mackintosh said: "Barbiturates are deadly easy, but easily dead."
(Fig. 2. 5)

2.2.2 Ketalar

No anaesthetic agent produced in the last 20 years has improved the anaesthetic situation so drastically as Ketalar, especially in developing countries. Ketalar is a powerful anaesthetic agent, offering a wide range of safety. Especially in up-country hospitals, where a single medical officer has to perform small or emergency operations and an anaesthetist or anaesthetic equipment is not available, Ketalar has a wide application. Ketalar is rapidly absorbed and an *acting* non-barbiturate general anaesthetic for IV and intramuscular (IM) use. It is metabolised by methylation and oxidation relatively quickly and excreted in the urine. Therapeutic doses of Ketalar produce a state of dissociation; a stupor-like sleep in which the patient usually has his eyes open. It is a strong analgetic with a weak hypnotic effect. In many cases the patient has unpleasant dreams and a sense of depersonalisation. This is markedly less the case in children.

2.2.2.1 Effects on the CVS

It is characteristic of Ketalar that after IV application there is a rise of BP. The maximum rise occurs after 3 min and this normalises after 10-20 min. According to my own experience the dosage does not influence in either way the increase of BP. In general there is a rise of systolic pressure by up to 26%, followed by diastolic pressure. There is a similar effect on the heart rate with an average rise of 28%-30% which takes the same time for normalisation.

2.2.2.2 Effects on the CRS

After quick IV application of the dosage, there can be a short lasting respiratory depression. Even after careful application there is a characteristic change in the respiratory rhythm. Some low-volume ventilation, followed by deep breathing with a volume up to 1500 cm^2 and increased saliva production. The blood gas analysis demonstrates that the respiration is sufficient, even after the change of rhythm. There is no evidence that dosages between 2-4 mg Ketalar/ kg body wt. can change the blood gas analysis, but from recent reports, the prevention of aspiration under Ketalar anaesthesia cannot be guaranteed.

2.2.2.3 Reflexes and Muscle Tonus

Reflexes for normal maintenance of the airway are usually present throughout. Generally there is no muscle relaxation and an increase in skeletal muscle tonus.

2.2.2.4 Laboratory Analysis

Until now major changes of the blood composition could not be detected. Of interest is the blood-sugar concentration: there is a rise of blood-sugar of about 10%-12% which should not inhibit the use of Ketalar for diabetic patients.

2.2.2.5 Dosage and Duration of Action

A normal IV dosage of 2 mg Ketalar/kg body wt. produces after a latence time of 30 s an anaesthesia lasting 5-15 min. Booster doses, if necessary, are 1 mg/ kg. Dosage of 5-10 mg Ketalar/kg given IM, produces anaesthesia lasting 20 min. The booster dose is half of the initial dosage.

2.2.2.6 Clinical Use of Ketalar

    a) As induction agent as a supplement to general anaesthesia
    b) Mono anaesthetic agent as single, repeated or as a drip

2.2.2.7 Disadvantages of Ketalar

It can be argued that the hypertensive effect of Ketalar should be considered a disadvantage. In many cases we have primarily to deal with hypotensive patients where the hypertensive effect is most welcome. The major disadvantages are: no relaxation (of consequence for abdominal surgery or where muscle relaxation is necessary); Ketalar anaesthesia can be associated with hallucination especially in the recovery period (premedication); finally, the drug is quite expensive.

2.2.2.8 Contraindications

    a) Any condition in which a rise of BP is undesirable
    b) Any condition in which a rise of pulse rate is undesirable
    c) Psychiatric patients
    d) Any condition in which a rise of intracranial pressure is undesirable

2.2.3 Propanidid (Epontol)

Propanidid is a short-acting hypnotic. The duration of action is 2-7 min with also a short post-anaesthetic period. It is very quickly metabolised in unspecific esters and eliminated by the kidneys. Propanidid passes the placenta only in significantly small amounts with no effect on the neonatal. The respiration in propanadid anaesthesia is very characteristic: after quick IV application the respiration starts with hyperventilation, which will gradually normalise (see Fig. 2.6). According to our experiences propanadid should be given at a rate of 10 ml or 0.5 g in 20-30 s. .

Epontol

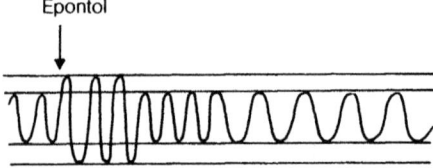

Fig. 2.6

The CVS does not show significant changes under low dosages. In older and wasted patients the dosage must be reduced to 5 mg propanidid/kg body wt. Recent reports show that there is frequently an allergy reaction towards the drug, so premedication with an antihistaminica is recommended.

2.3 Neuromuscular Blocking Drugs

These are drugs that paralyse muscles voluntarily and they are used primarily as adjunctive agents during anaesthesia. According to their action muscle relaxants are divided into two groups:

(1) Non-depolarising agents, e.g. tubocurarine and the synthetics and
(2) Depolarising agents, e.g. succinyl-bi-choline

The action of neither agent does not take place on the muscle or on the nerves. *They act on the so-called end-plate, the space between the muscle and the nerve.*

The neuromuscular blocking drugs are quaternary aminos and not suitable for oral administration. They are well-absorbed IV. Succinyl-bi-choline can be given diluted IM in 0.2% solution to children. Non-depolarising agents are usually fixed to the plasma, while their metabolic fate is not yet quite known. 40-80% is excreted unchanged by the kidneys. Succinyl-bi-choline is hydrolysed step wise by pseudocholinesterase to succinyl mono-choline, succinate and choline. In a normal transmission of a nerve impulse and muscle movement, an impulse of the nerve reaches the end-plate, the transmitter acetylcholine (A-Ch) is released and reaches the muscle receptor. This causes depolarisation, e.g. exchange of electrolysis and contraction of the muscles. In a few seconds, the A-Ch is metabolised by a ferment called cholinesterase. The electric exchange drops, the muscle falls in its resting position and a new impulse can be expected.

2.3.1 Non-depolarising Muscle Relaxant

The non-depolarising agents act at the muscle end-plate and prevent A-Ch from exerting its action. *The action is purely one of blocking.* A-Ch is still liberated, but in the presence of the blocking agent, depolarisation of the receptor does not take place. After the IV administration muscle weakness or flaccid paralysis (depending upon the dosage) begins after 3 min and maximum effect is reached within 5 min. First affected are muscles of the neck and eyes (the eyelids drop and the patient has difficulty in speaking); other small muscles such as those of the hands and legs are followed by abdomen, chest and finally the diaphragm.

This condition can be overcome by an increase of A-Ch. The concentration of A-Ch can increase: (a) if enough time elapses for A-Ch to be built up and the non-depolarisation agent is taken away by the plasma or (b) by the administration of a cholinesterase inhibitor such as neostigmine.

The non-depolarisation agent can be reversed by a cholinesterase inhibitor, which, however, stimulates the parasympathetic vagus, causing bradycardia broncho-secretion, vasodilation and fall of BP. All this is increased in the case of high CO_2. This effect can be counteracted by a vagolytic-like atropine. For reversing, neostigmine should always be given together with atropine: 0.01 mg atropine/kg body wt., 0.02 mg neostigmine/kg body wt. (0.08 for children) or 1.0 mg neostigmine per 10 mg curarine. At least 5 min elapse until the full action of neostigmine takes place; after the administration of neostigmine the patient has to be ventilated up until full respiration is restored. Non-depolarising relaxants like tubocurarine have a weak sympathetic ganglia blocking effect, which may result in a fall of BP. This can be remarkable in halothane anaesthesia. There is also a slight histamine-releasing effect.

2.3.1.1 Dosage and Duration of Action

Non-depolarising relaxants are mainly long-acting.

Tubarine

Dosage: 0.2-0.3 mg/kg body wt.
Duration: 20-40 min
Repeated dosage: 0.08-1.0 mg/kg body wt.

Gallamine (Flaxedil) is a synthetic, non-depolarising relaxant, causing tachycardia and occasionally rise of BP. It is entirely excreted by the kidneys (80%) and crosses the placenta. This agent therefore should be avoided:

a) In kidney disease
b) In C.S.= sectio caesarea
c) In patients where a rise of pulse rate is harmful

Dosage: 1-2 mg Flaxedil/kg body wt.
Duration: 20-30 min

Alloferin has fewer side-effects than tubarine, no histamine liberation and less ganglia blocking effect.

Dosage: 0.1-0.2 mg Alloferin/kg body wt.
Duration: 15-20 min

Pankuronium has also a few side-effects but long duration of action. It is thermo-unstable and must be kept in the refrigerator.

2.3.2 Depolarising Relaxant (Succinyl-bi-choline)

The agent acts like A-Ch. It causes self-depolarisation.
    When A-Ch arrives, the depolarisation has already taken place. No impulses can be transmitted. This complete depolarisation after IV application leads to inco-ordinated contraction of the muscles, which is followed by complete relaxation after 30 s. The body, however, is able to produce a ferment called pseudocholinesterase in a period of 3-4 min, which breaks down succinyl-bi-choline (S-Ch) and the action is over. We have herewith a short-acting muscle relaxant. After IV application there is a rise of K^+ in the serum causing, especially in the heart, bradycardia and arrythmia. S-Ch has to be used carefully in patients with burns, up to 6-8 weeks after the burn. If S-Ch is used for a longer time, e.g. succinyl drip, doses over 500 mg can lead to a dual block.
    Generally, succinyl has no histamine liberation property, passes the placenta quickly, but is very quickly metabolised in the foetus so that use of succinyl in obstetric anaesthesia is not contraindicated.

Dosage: 1 mg succinyl/kg body wt. (but no more than 8 mg/kg in a drip)
Duration: 3-8 min

    Muscle relaxants are mainly used as adjunctives in combination anaesthesia to achieve muscle relaxation while the anaesthetic is kept very light. Long acting muscle relaxants are also used for relaxation and artificial respiration in tetanus patients. Succinyl is mainly used for induction and intubation of anaesthesia.

Table 2.5. Summary

Drug	Ons. of act.	Dur. of act.	Mode of act.	C.V.S.	R.S.
Scoline	i.v. 20 s i.m. 1-2 min	Short 4-7 min -20 min	Depolarisation	Bradycardia	Apnea ◙
d.Tubocurin	3 min	Long 30-60 min	Compl. block of Acetylcholine	Fall of B P	Apnea ◙
Alloferin	2 min	20-40 min	,,	–	Apnea ◙
Gallamin (Flaxedil)	1-2 min	20-40 min	,,	Tachycardia	Apnea ◙
Pavulon (Pankuronium)	2 min	-60 min	,,	–	Apnea ◙

Drug	Dosage	Antagonists	
Scoline	1 mg/kg	Ө	
d.Tubocurin	0.2 mg/kg	Neostigmin/atropine	
Alloferin	0.1 mg/kg	,,	,,
Gallamin (Flaxedil)	2 mg/kg	,,	,,
Pavulon (Pankuronium)	0.02 mg/kg	,,	,,

◙ = Due to muscle relaxation

2.4 Other Drugs Used in Anaesthesia

2.4.1 Atropine

Atropine is extracted from a shrub called *Atropa belladonna* and is available in amounts of 0.5 mg, ml or tablets. Atropine and all related drugs prohibit nerve impulses at the post-ganglionic nerve-ending where A-Ch is the transmitter. In this way atropine lowers the action of the parasympathetic nervous system, which results in:

    a) Pupillary dilatation
    b) Reduction of the gland production (saliva by mouth and bronchia)
    c) Increase of pulse rate
    d) Dilatation of bronchial trees

Since most drugs have a parasympathetic effect there is a possibility of vagal reflexes, e.g. bradycardia, arrythmia and increased saliva production. *Premedication with atropine is essential.* For premedication atropine is given IM 30-40 min before anaesthesia begins. For adults the dosage is 0.1 mg atropine/10 kg body wt. The recommended dosage for children is:

age + 2 : 20 = mg

3 J. + 2 = 5 : 20 = 0.25 mg

If for any reasons IM application is not possible, half of the IM dosage can be given intravenously, at least 5 min before anaesthesia is started.

2.4.2 Analgetica

To reduce pain, intensive analgetica are used for premedication together with atropine. Morphine and other naturally occurring narcotica and their semisynthetic modifications are isolated from opium, which is collected from one special variety of poppy *(Papaver somniferum)*.

2.4.2.1 Mechanism of Action

The effects of morphine and related drugs are due to a mixture of depression on some specific CNS functions and stimulation of others and of a mixture of sympathomimetic and parasympathomimetic influence (see Fig. 2.7).

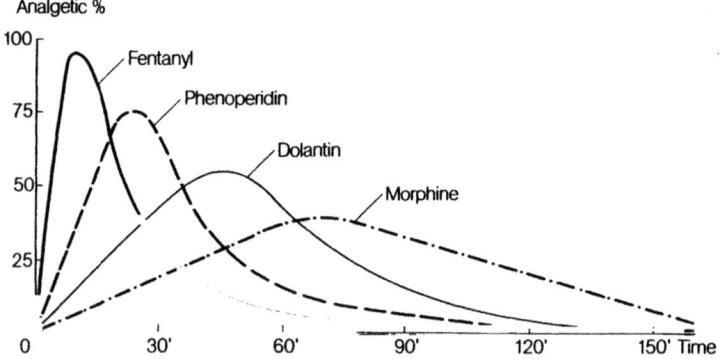

Fig. 2.7 (from Stöcker, Narkose. Georg Thieme Verlag, Stuttgart 4th ed., 1976)

2.4.2.2 Effects of Analgetics

The essential pharmacological effect of the strong analgetics is the relief of pain. Pain is said to involve two components: (1) the sensation reaching the CNS and (2) the individual psychical process and reaction. Morphine alters the second of these processes and the patient may report that the pain is still present but less distressing. The narcotic analgesic relief of pain is universal, almost regardless of its origin or intensity. Under smaller dosages, patients are quite relaxed but still responsive. From increasingly larger doses the patient will become drowsy, inattentive and inefficient and falls into a sleep from which he may still be aroused. Very large doses induce coma.

The sensitivity of medullary centres to CO_2 and the respiration is correspondingly depressed. Nausea and vomiting are caused by a stimulating action of morphine on the chemoreceptive trigger in the CNS. It has been demonstrated that morphine is a histamine liberator: this action can explain itching and urticaria which may appear.

The heart rate and cardial output are slowed and reduced only by larger doses, but morphine has a hypotensive effect which can cause dizziness or fainting. The skin is warm and flushed. All of the opiates and synthetic equivalents are well absorbed from the site of administration and metabolised mainly in the liver. Due to the *sedative and pain reducing effect*, morphine and its relatives are used in anaesthesia for premedication and post-operative treatment of pain.

2.4.2.3 Dosages of the Different Agents

Morphine is mostly given subcutaneously: 10-15 mg in adults

Oral dose: 8-20 mg morphine in adults
Duration: 4-8 h

Pethedine is less potent than morphine but causes also less respiratory depression.

Dosage: 2 mg Pethedine/kg body wt.
Duration: 4-6 h

Fetanyl is a new, synthetic, strong analgetic with a short duration of action mainly used in neuroleptic anaesthesia.

2.4.3 Narcotic Antagonists

The antagonists exert narcotic action by the same mechanism as morphine. The relation is competitive and the action is explained by the displacement of the agonist from the receptor.

Nalorphine Dosage: 2-4 mg or 0.1 mg/kg body wt. given IV as initial dosage, which can be repeated after 2-3 h.

2.4.4 Neuroleptica

Droperidol and haloperidol are so-called neuroleptica and can be strongly differentiated from the hypnotica in their effect. Patients are in a tranquil state without any subjective feeling of sedation. Under normal dosages there is very little depressing effect on the CRS and the CVS. After good premedication with haloperidol there is generally a fall of B P by 10% caused by the alpha receptor-blocking action of the drug. There is, however, very little effect on the pulse rate. There is also a strong anti-memetic effect, an advantage in ether anaesthesia. In high or over-dosages it may produce extra-pyramidal excitement and irritation. The advantages of neuroleptica are:

a) Low toxicity
b) Stable circulation
c) Strong anti-emetic effect
d) Good tranquilising effect

Haloperidol

Dosage: 0.2 mg/kg body wt. 1-1 1/2 h pre-operative
Duration: 8-10 h

Droperidol

Dosage: 0.3 mg/kg body wt.
Duration: 6-8 h

2.4.5 Diazepam (Valium)

A potent transquiliser and effective in relieving pre-operative anxiety, Valium is a very well-known drug with a good sedative and muscle relaxing effect.

Large doses cause drowsiness and unconsciousness, though their toxicity is relatively low. Dosage: 0.2 mg Valium/kg body wt.

2.4.6 Tranquilisers (Promethazine)

The manifest effect of the tranquiliser is depression in the sense of reduced activity and attentiveness. As larger doses are given, signs of stimulation appear. Promethazine has atropine-like properties, is parasympathetic and has antihistamine as well as anti-emetic effects. It is mainly used for premedication. Dosage: 0.5-1 mg/kg body wt. IM or IV.

2.5 List of Drugs Commonly Used in Anaesthesia

1) Atropine 0.5 mg ampoules
2) Diazepam 10 mg ampoules and tablets
3) Droperidol or haloperidol, ampoules and tablets
4) Ether 250 ml bottles
5) Epontol 0.5 g ampoules
6) Gallamine 80 mg ampoules
7) Halothane 250 ml bottles
8) Ketalar 50 mg/ml, 10 ml vial
9) Morphine 10 mg ampoules
10) Neostigmine 0.5 mg and 2.5 mg ampoules
11) Pancuronium 4 mg ampoules
12) Pethedine 100 mg ampoules
13) Suxamethonium (Sooline) 100 mg vial
14) Tubocurarine 15 mg ampoules
15) Thiopentone 0.5 g ampoules

Chapter 3
Pre-operative Examination

The possibility of performing adequate anaesthesia largely depends upon pre-operative examination and evaluation of the patient. The anaesthetist must know his patient and co-ordinate this knowledge with his strategy in using drugs and methods for performing anaesthesia. It is equally important that the patient knows his anaesthetist and has confidence in him. Pre-anaesthetic visits and examinations are therefore essential for routine work. Use of a fixed schedule as follows or an anaesthetic protocol helps to achieve a systematic pre-operative examination. Make sure it is the right patient and know the weight length and age. A picture of the patient's condition can be evaluated through:

1) Patient's history
2) Clinical examination
3) Laboratory investigations

3.1 History of the patient (see Table 3.1)

3.2 Clinical Examination

3.3 Laboratory Investigations

3.4 Summary

Pre-anaesthetic examination helps to establish an over-all picture of the patient, according to which he can be put into one of the five following classifications for anaesthesia:

Table 3.1

History of the patient

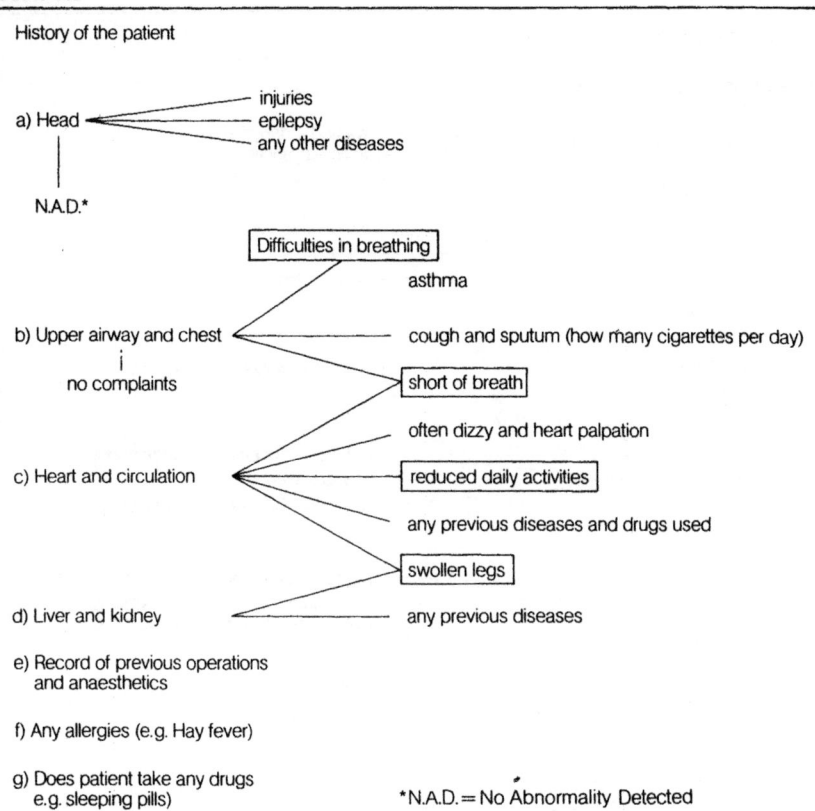

a) Head — injuries
— epilepsy
— any other diseases

N.A.D.*

Difficulties in breathing
asthma

b) Upper airway and chest — cough and sputum (how many cigarettes per day)
no complaints — short of breath

often dizzy and heart palpation

c) Heart and circulation — reduced daily activities

any previous diseases and drugs used

swollen legs

d) Liver and kidney — any previous diseases

e) Record of previous operations and anaesthetics

f) Any allergies (e.g. Hay fever)

g) Does patient take any drugs e.g. sleeping pills)

*N.A.D. = No Abnormality Detected

1) Normal healthy patient (aside from his surgical problems)
2) Patient with mild systemic diseases, 11.5 g % Hgb., slight cough and hypo- or hypertension *is considered fit for anaesthesia.*
3) Patient with severe systemic disease that limits activity; Hgb. less than 10 g% pure bronchitis; beginning C.C.F., *needs treatment first.*
4) Patient with an incapacitating systemic disease which is a threat to life: C.C.F., shock, severe lung insufficiency, etc., is in a *very poor condition for anaesthesia.* Energetic treatment indicated.
5) Moribund patient where death is to be expected.

Nevertheless, there are situations calling for emergency surgical treatment: bleeding peptic ulcer, intussusception etc. In such cases surgery is prior to the treatment of the other problems. These cases call for emergency anaesthesia and the anaesthetic strategy has to be adapted to the needs of the situation.

Table 3.1 (continued)

Clinical examination

a) General impression of patient

    1. Physical: —————————— wasted – dehydrated
          | toxic – cyanotic
    Fit and healthy

                                semiconscious
    2. Mental: —————————— confused
         | nervous, frightened
    Quiet – relaxed

b) Head and Eyes ——————————— any signs of jaundice, anaemia
   |
   N.A.D.

                              can patient open mouth wide enough
c) Upper Airway ——————————— any loose teeth
   | any tumour in mouth and neck region
   N.A.D.

                            Mode of respiration: frequency and depth
d) Lungs ————————————————— comfortable breathing while lying flat
                              (can count up to 15 in a single breath)

                               clear
    Stethoscope – both lungs
                               squeezing conception
                               crepitations

| If history of chest disease: X-ray of chest essential! |

                              blood pressure
                                              frequency
                              pulse
                                              rhythm
e) Heart and circulation
                              size of heart (X-ray?)
                              oedema – ascites – hepatomegaly
                              signs of cyanosis

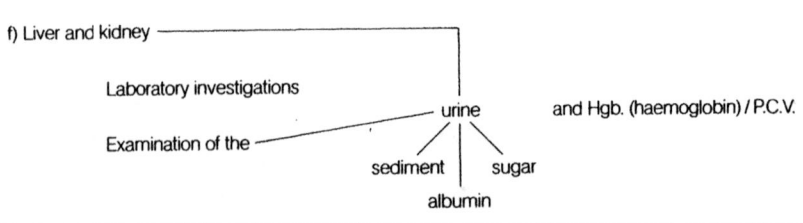

f) Liver and kidney

    Laboratory investigations

                             urine   and Hgb. (haemoglobin) / P.C.V.
    Examination of the
                      sediment | sugar
                           albumin

3.5 Comments

A fit and healthy patient who presents no major complaints besides his surgical problems is fit for anaesthesia and is even competent to compensate the side-effects of anaesthesia. An old and wasted patient has a low metabolic rate and therefore anaesthetic drugs have to be reduced by half. If there are any signs of dehydration patients should be rehydrated first. Rehydration during anaesthesia is difficult or even impossible.

3.6.1 Cyanosis

Cyanotic patients are in *great danger*. Reasons for cyanosis must be found and if possible treated first. If there is any doubt as to the mental condition of the patient, look for the reasons first, thinking of the following possibilities:

a) Drugs
b) Diabetes
c) Uraemia
d) Typhoid fever
e) Mental disease

A confused patient, if you do not know the reasons, is unfit for routine anaesthesia.

A nervous patient requires good premedication. In case of a history of head injuries or epilepsy try to avoid anaesthetic drugs which increase intracranial pressure, like Scoline or Ketalar.

3.6.2 Tumours etc.

In the case of tumours, stenosis and inability to open the mouth wide enough, careful examination and preparation has to be carried out, until the anaesthetist is absolutely sure he can maintain the airway during operation (see Chap. 5). In such a situation local or Ketalar anaesthesia is preferable; also make sure a tracheostomy set (or tray) is available.

3.6.3 Lung Disease

Except for emergencies give no anaesthesia where lung disease is present!

A slight cough but clear lungs does not hinder anaesthesia, provided there is good post-operative care. Chest diseases with cough, wet chest and temperature, contraindicate routine anaesthesia. Patients should first be treated with expectorants, breathing excercises and antibiotics. If there is a history of any chest disease and doubt about the condition of the lungs and heart, an X-ray picture of the chest is important and examination of the sputum is essential. In the case of an emergency operation, local Ketalar or a slight general anaesthesia with muscle relaxants is indicated.

The asthma patient needs good premedication: promethazine, aminophylline or hydrocortisone. For anaesthesia avoid drugs with a notable histamine liberating effect, like curarine. Remember that asthma patients are often allergic to drugs.

3.6.4 Circulation Problems

Difficulty in breathing while lying flat is a sign of left-side heart failure. Patients with C.C.F. (Congestive Cardiac Failure) dysponoea, oedema or an enlarged liver are unfit for routine anaesthesia or at least, poor candidates. Such patients need medical treatment first.

Cases of compensated heart disease (reduced daily activity, but adequate B P, dyspnoea only by exercise but no oedema) should not present great problems, but you should observe the following points:

a) Maintenance of good O_2 tension during anaesthesia
b) Avoid hypotension
c) Careful replacement of blood loss
d) Adequate fluid and electrolyte replacement (careful)

3.6.5 Hypotension

Hypotension due to heart failure, anaemia or volume deficit should be treated first. Hypotension in vagotonic patients usually does not present great problems; good premedication, preferably with neuroleptica, is advised.

3.6.6 Hypertension

Induction of anaesthesia may produce severe hypertension; therefore induction has to be slow. Small doses of thiopentone are recommended. Ketalar is contraindicated because of its hypertensive action. Hypertensive drugs given before the operation can lead to a serious fall of BP during anaesthesia.

3.6.7 Arrhythmia

Arrhythmia is a sign of C.C.F., heart disease or an anaemic murmur which disappears after treatment. Murmurs without other complaints or pathological signs do not present contraindications for anaesthesia.

3.6.8 Tachycardia

Heart failure, volume deficit or associated with pyrexia (temperature)

3.6.9 Bradycardia

Digitalisation (sportsman's pulse).

3.6.10 Hepatomegaly and Ascites

Hepatomegaly and ascites are indications of either C.C.F. or active lung disease. All anaesthetic drugs more or less depress the liver function and are partly metabolised in the liver. In the case of present liver disease, selective surgery should be avoided. However, if an operation is essential use local anaesthesia or reduce the dosage of general anaesthetic drugs by half. Patients with liver disease may be resistant to curare, but sensitive to suxamethonium (succinylcholine).

3.6.11 Temperature

A high temperature indicates a disease and investigations have to be carried out first to find the origin of the temperature. Anaesthesia may be given in emergencies only. Patients with pyrexia have a high metabolic rate and therefore require more O_2 and fluids.

3.6.12 History of Drug Taking

Patients who have been on prolonged steroid therapy should be considered as special anaesthetic risks. The treatment should be stopped a long time before anaesthesia or supplementary steroid therapy is to be given. (surgical problem.) Patients who have been taking any sedatives for a long time will be affected in one way or another. Patients who receive phenothiazine derivatives may be sensitive to barbiturates with marked hypotension and a prolonged recovery period, while patients who take barbiturates or are used to alcohol are quite resistant to barbiturates.

3.7 Laboratory Investigation

No anaesthesia should be administered without examination of haemoglobin (Hgb.) and urine, especially in dehydrated patients. Hgb. or P.C.V. are necessary to estimate the degree of haemoconcentration. Hgb. concentrations of 11 g% are adequate for anaesthesia, but below 10 g%, patients are poor candidates for surgery and if possible the haemoglobin level should be raised first by iron in non-urgent cases or by transfusion in urgent cases. If urine shows positive sugar further investigation and treatment are indicated first. In the case of positive albumin and oedema: general anaesthetic is contraindicated.

3.8 Remember

No (routine) anaesthesia in the full presence of lung disease is recommended, or where you are not sure you can maintain ventilation. Low haemoglobin and inadequate functioning of heart and circulation need treatment first, although in an emergency this can be done in a matter of hours.

On the satisfactory function of the liver and kidneys depends the patient's ability to break down and excrete the majority of anaesthetics. The sicker the patient and the older, the less drugs he needs. No barbiturates should be given in kidney disease.

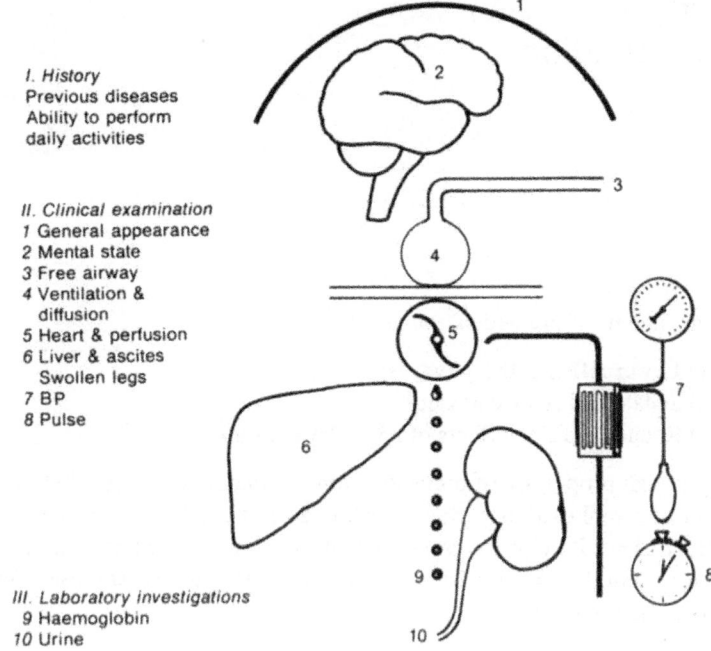

I. History
Previous diseases
Ability to perform
daily activities

II. Clinical examination
1 General appearance
2 Mental state
3 Free airway
4 Ventilation &
   diffusion
5 Heart & perfusion
6 Liver & ascites
   Swollen legs
7 BP
8 Pulse

III. Laboratory investigations
9 Haemoglobin
10 Urine

Fig. 3.1. Summary

Chapter 4
Premedication

The main aims of premedication are to:

1) Lower reflex activity (vagus)
2) Sedate and reduce anxiety
3) Reduce the side-effects of anaesthetic drugs

Through proper use of premedication the quantity of anaesthetics *and* the danger of complications during anaesthesia can be reduced. It makes it easier for the patient; it helps to disperse his fears and worries while waiting for his operation and it makes it easier for the anaesthetist to anaesthetise a relaxed and confident patient.

4.1 Lowering of Reflex Activity

Most anaesthetica *stimulate* the parasympathetiç activity, causing broncho-secretion, bronchospasm, bradycardia and fall of B P. Therefore *premedicate with vagolytica like atropine.* Atropine lowers parasympathetic activity, causing drying of the respiratory tract, tachycardia. In this way it not only counteracts the side-effects of some anaesthetic drugs but also provides a more favourable situation for anaesthesia.

Dosage: 0.01 mg atropine/kg body wt. IM at least 20-30 min before operation or IV at least 5-7 min before operation.

Contraindication: all cases where an increase of pulse rate is contraindicated, e.g. thyrotoxicosis, digitalised patients and in glaucoma. In these cases a tranquiliser like promethazine can be used which has, aside from tranquilising, a vagolytic effect (see Chap. 2).

4.2 Sedation and Reduction of Anxiety

For this purpose the vagolytics can be combined with:

1) Neuroleptics
2) Sedatives and analgesics
3) Tranquilisers

4.2.1 Neuroleptics

For routine premedication where *no* severe pain exists, neuroleptica are commonly used because of their low toxicity, their good tranquilising and anti-emetic effect, reducing the side-effects of anaesthetic drugs, e.g. vomiting after ether anaesthesia. Neuroleptics have a slight alphareceptor blocking action, which results in a slight fall of BP (10%) after premedication.

Dehydrobenzperidol (DHB): 0.3 mg/kg body wt. IM or IV 1 h pre-operatively. Haloperidol: 0.1 mg/kg/body wt. IM or per os 1-2 h before operation. Since haloperidol is a good tranquiliser and anti-emetic but with poor sedative effect it can be combined with nitrazepam (Mogadon): 0.2 mg/kg per os. As both drugs can be administered orally and have a middle long duration of action, the premedication can easily be given to the patient in the ward even when the time of operation is not definitely settled. In this case the vagolytics can be given together with the induction agent e.g. Penthotal.

A wide range of premedication has been tried in an attempt to control the hallucination after Ketalar anaesthesia. Premedication with neuroleptics, and atropine, where Ketalar was used as an anaesthetic drug, has shown promising results.

4.2.2 Sedative Analgesics

Pethedine and morphia are commonly used in patients where, besides sedation, reduction of pain is needed. These will also reduce the level of pain sensitivity during anaesthesia, an advantage when for maintaining anaesthesia, an anaesthetic agent with poor analgesic effect is used. Dosage:

Pethedine: 1-2 mg/kg body wt. IM, 30 min before operation (IV not recommended)
Morphia: 0.2 mg/kg body wt. IM only, 30-60 min pre-operatively.

4.2.3 Tranquiliser

Promethazine is mainly used in addition to pethedine or where atropine is contraindicated. Promethazine potentiates the action of pethedine; therefore the dosage of pethedine is to be deduced to 1 mg/kg body wt. Where an antihistaminic effect for premedication is wanted, e.g. in asthma patients

Dosage: 1 mg/kg body wt. IM or IV.

4.3 Premedication for Children and Infants

Children under two years usually do not require premedication. They do not understand or experience anxiety, but to avoid crying while being brought into the operating room, premedication with neuroleptics is suitable. Atropine is essential.

Dosage: 0-6 months 0.3 mg atropine IM
           6-18 months 0.4 mg atropine IM
           2 years 0.5 mg atropine IM
over   2 years 0.5 mg atropine IM

For relief of pain and sedation: 1-2 mg pethedine/kg body wt. IM. Neuroleptics are successfully administered orally, an advantage in children, because of their fear of injection.

0.1 mg haloperidol drops/kg body wt. + 0.2 mg Mogadon/kg body wt. per os 1 h before operation.

4.4 Summary

The dosage of premedication depends on the body weight, age and the general condition of the patient. The older the patient, the lower the metabolic rate and the slower the metabolism of the drugs, which means lowering the dosage (see Fig. 4.1). The operation is to be performed at the peak of the pharmacological action of the pre-anaesthetic drug. Therefore the right time for premedication must be carefully considered.

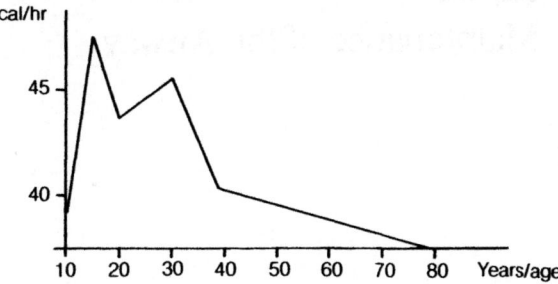

Fig. 4.1. Metabolic rate/age

Chapter 5

Maintenance of the Airway

The responsibility of the anaesthetist is to keep the patient alive and free of pain during surgery. The success, however, largely depends on the ability to maintain the airway with adequate gas exchange during anaesthesia. The anatomical airway lies between the lips and nostrils and the alveoli of the lungs. (During anaesthesia it lies between the source of fresh air or gas and the alveoli.) It is important to know all the possible sources of obstruction and to have the qualification to master them. The prevention of respiratory obstruction begins with pre-operative examination (see Chap. 3) and the preparation of all the necessary technical equipment. Obstruction of the airway will, after a short time, lead to asphyxia and the condition will deteriorate rapidly and finally to cardiac arrest (see Figs. 5.1 and 5.2). *Never put a patient to sleep when you are not absolutely sure you can maintain the airway.*

Consequence of insufficient ventilation of respiratory obstruction

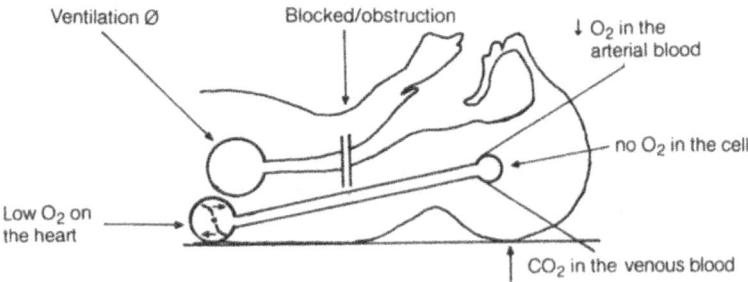

Fig. 5.1

Signs of respiratory obstruction are:

    a) Breathing sounds are noisy or absent
    b) Cyanosis (tongue, blood, finger tips)
    c) Chest movements are diminished or paradoxical

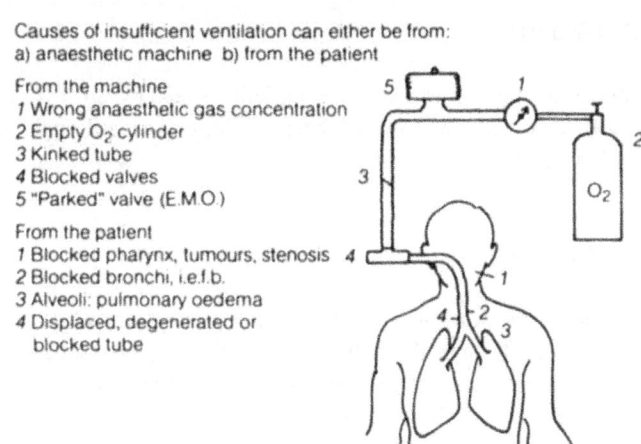

Causes of insufficient ventilation can either be from:
a) anaesthetic machine b) from the patient

From the machine
1 Wrong anaesthetic gas concentration
2 Empty O_2 cylinder
3 Kinked tube
4 Blocked valves
5 "Parked" valve (E.M.O.)

From the patient
1 Blocked pharynx, tumours, stenosis
2 Blocked bronchi, i.e.f.b.
3 Alveoli: pulmonary oedema
4 Displaced, degenerated or
   blocked tube

Conclusion

One of the major concerns of the anaesthetist is the maintenance of an adequate airway and gas exchange. It is therefore important to know all the possible sources of obstruction and to have the qualification to master them. The prevention of respiratory obstruction begins already with pre-operative examination (see Chap. 3) and the preparation of all technical equipment necessary.

5.1 Causes of Respiratory Obstruction in the Patient

5.1.1 Loose Teeth

Before anaesthesia, make sure that there are no loose teeth or any foreign bodies in the mouth, for both can cause severe respiratory obstruction. Furthermore, you want to make sure that the patient can open his mouth wide enough.

5.1.2 Tumours

Complete obstruction under deep anaesthesia or in a relaxed patient can be caused by tumours. If anaesthesia has to be performed all kinds of endotracheal tubes and equipment should be available and everything ready for immediate tracheotomy. Pre-operative signs of obstruction may even be an indication for tracheotomy as a necessary preparation for anaesthesia.

5.1.3 Stenosis

Stenosis is unlikely to worsen in patients asleep except for difficulties in intubation. Thin tubes and introducers are important, although these cases are best left to experts.

5.1.4 Pharynx

The most common cause of obstruction in a patient who is not intubated is the pharynx, though the falling back of the tongue is a danger in every patient who is unconscious and relaxed and lying on his back. Respiration will be snoring and insufficient (see Fig. 5.3 and 5.4).

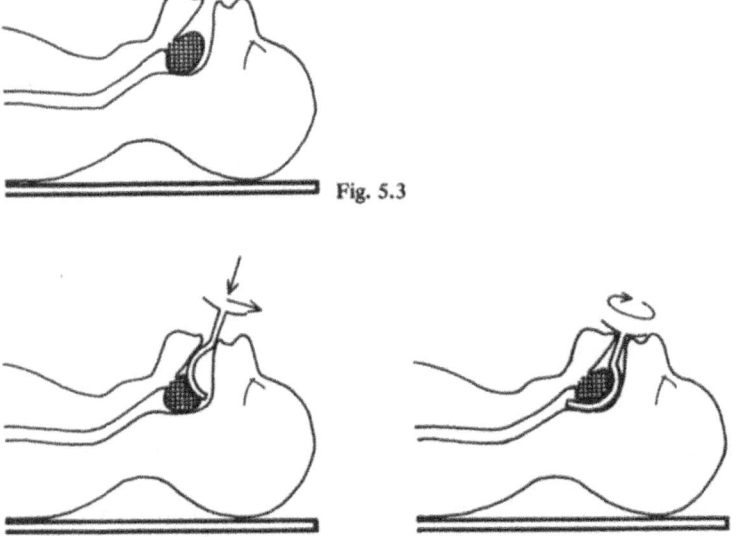

Fig. 5.3

Fig. 5.4

An airway is only fulfilling its function when there is no longer a pharyngeal reflex, otherwise it may provoke vomiting.

5.1.5 Vomiting

The greatest hazard in anaesthesia, which can easily cost the life of the patient, is vomiting. The best safeguard is an empty stomach but unfortunately there is no way of telling that the stomach is completely empty. Aspiration obstruction of the airway can appear either through: (1) active vomiting or (2) passive regurgitation. Vomiting during induction with penthotal-ether when the laryngeal reflex is still present may easily result in laryngeal spasm and consequently anoxia and further complications. Regurgitation in deep anaesthesia where the laryngeal reflex is relaxed can occur unnoticed. Wet breath, sounds, rattling and cyanosis indicate the beginning of the catastrophy. *The best prevention of aspiration obstruction is intubation.* There is always a danger of aspiration in deep anaesthesia without intubation. If vomiting occurs: head down position, head to the side and clean the airway with a sucker.

5.1.6 Spasm

Laryngeal or broncho-spasms arise from irritation of the cords caused by:

a) Strong vapour irritants
b) Aspiration, vomitus, saliva
c) Reflex spasm from the operation (vagus)

If a spasm occurs, stop anaesthesia. Clean the airway, give O_2, and relax the patient with Scoline followed by intubation, ventilation and bronchial toilet.

5.1.7 Obstruction of the Trachea and Bronchi

Profuse secretion or sputum may flood the bronchial tree. Vomit or a foreign body may block smaller or bigger bronchial branches. Premedication with atropine, frequent sucking, and possibly intubation and intertracheal sucking may be necessary. If there is pulmonary oedema (as in heart failure) leading to impaired diffusion and poor gas exchange across the alveolar wall, then give no anaesthesia until after the condition has been corrected by O_2, diuretica and digoxine. *There is always a real possibility of inadequate ventilation during anaesthesia. Endotracheal intubation is one of the best ways of maintaining O_2 tension during anaesthesia.*

5.2 Intubation

5.2.1 Indications and Contraindications

5.2.1.1 Poor-Risk Patients

Where insufficient respiration and circulation are already present, the depressing effect of the anaesthetic will worsen the condition drastically and lead to major complications. Intubation and assisted or controlled ventilation is indicated in these cases to ensure good O_2 tension.

5.2.1.2 Operations on Certain Parts of the Body

In operations on the head, face, neck, thorax and upper abdomen intubation is obligatory.

5.2.1.3 Position of the Patient

Intubation is required in operations where the patient is to be placed in any unphysiological position, e.g. face down.

5.2.1.4 Severity and Length of the Operation

For all big operations the patient should be intubated to ensure adequate ventilation over a long period and reduce dead space.

5.2.1.5 Contraindication

Actually there is no contraindication to intubation, except for technical reasons where the necessary equipment is not available. However, the danger of inaccuracies during intubation should be kept in mind.

5.2.2 Technical Equipment

1) Endotracheal tubes and adapters
2) Laryngoscope
3) Source for Intermittant Positive Pressure Respiration (I.P.P.R.), e.g. Ambu-bag

5.2.2.1 Endotracheal Tubes

There are different types of endotracheal tubes made of rubber or plastic (see Fig. 5.5). Cuffed tubes have a thin-wall inflatable cuff, designed to lie immedi-

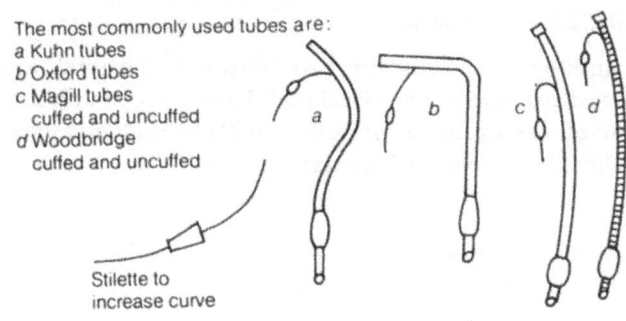

The most commonly used tubes are:
a Kuhn tubes
b Oxford tubes
c Magill tubes
   cuffed and uncuffed
d Woodbridge
   cuffed and uncuffed

Stilette to
increase curve

Fig. 5.5

ately below the cords. This seals the trachea and prevents both foreign material from entering the tracheal tree and the escape of anaesthetic gas from around the tube when the patient is artificially ventilated. The cuff is inflated via a rubber tube running along the tracheal catheter (see Fig. 5.6). Inflate the cuff until just airtight — more can cause ischaemia on the tracheal wall.

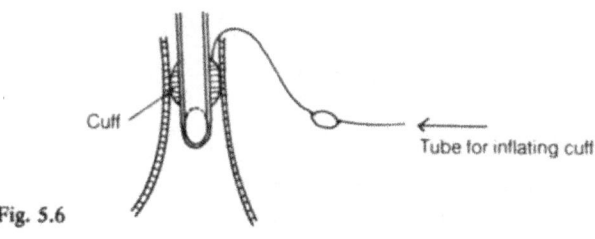

Cuff

Tube for inflating cuff

Fig. 5.6

Table 5.1. Sizes of endotracheal tubes: Twice the distance between the ear lobe and the corner of the mouth gives a rough guide of the length of tube required for oral intubation. *This table gives a guide for the correct diameter of the tube!*

Age	B W /kg	diam./mm	cm length	Magill	Systems
−6 mo		2.5-3.5	10-11.5	00-0	T-piece/E. valve Ambu
−1 yr	−10	−4.5	12-13	1	,,
1-3 yrs	−15	4.5-5.5	14	2-3	,,
3-6 yrs	−20	−6.5	16	3-4	half open
6-9 yrs	−22	6.5	18	5	,,
9-12 yrs	−30	7	20	6	,,
14-16 yrs		7	22	7	,,

Adult female size: 8   male size: 9

5.2.2.2 Laryngoscope

Anaesthetic laryngoscopes have batteries in the handle and a light source. The most common are the Mackintosh Laryngoscope with a bent blade and the Magill Laryngoscope with a straight blade. Both have exchangeable blades for children, normal and large sizes (see Fig. 5.7).

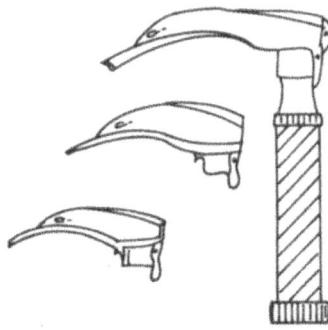

Fig. 5.7

5.2.3 Methods of Intubation

Intubation may be:

    a) Oral (through the mouth)
    b) Nasal (through the nostril)

For intubation to be performed, the reflexes must be absent:

    a) In light anaesthesia with muscle relaxation
    b) In deep anaesthesia
    c) In local anaesthesia

5.2.4 Oral Intubation under Light Anaesthesia with Muscular Relaxation

1. *Make sure that everything is ready for intubation:*

a) Laryngoscope (check whether the light is working!)
b) Endotracheal tubes (different sizes)
c) Syringe for blocking the cuff (inflating the cuff)
d) Small artery forceps (for clamping the cuff's tube)
e) Airway
f) Connector

g) Local anaesthesia spray if required
h) Magill's forceps
i) Plaster
k) Apparatus for ventilation

2. Put head of patient on a cushion of 4 inches, so as to get the correct angle between mouth-epiglottis-trachea.

3. *Induction* of anaesthesia and relaxation followed by inhalation of O_2 air via a mask until apnoea is achieved.

4. As soon as *apnoea and areflexia* are reached, stretch the head in the so-called Jackson position (see Fig. 5.8).

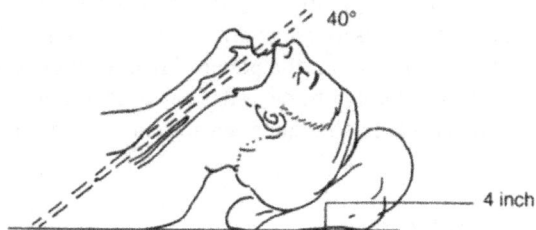

Fig. 5.8. Jackson position

5. Open the mouth with the thumb and the first finger of the *right* hand, hold the *laryngoscope* in the *left* hand and slide the blade into the right side of the mouth, pushing the tongue side- and downward, until the epiglotis is seen. Place the curved (Mackintosh) blade above the epiglottis and lift upward to expose the larynx. Do not press on the upper teeth (Fig. 5.9).

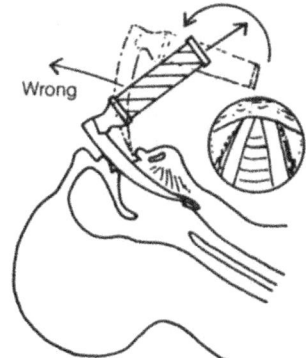

Fig. 5.9

6. Induce the *endotracheal tube* gently into the visible tracheal opening, so that the cuff lies below the vocal cords. One way to check if the tube is in the trachea is to press with the left hand on the chest. If the tube is in the right place, air will come out as you press. *Never use force.*

7. Hold the tube with the left hand, connect the tube with the *bellows* (with the help of a second person), ventilate and check if both lungs are ventilated. Blow up the cuff and fix the tube with the help of a plaster.

8. Put the head in the right position, check both lungs again and continue with I.P.P.R.

As there is danger of spreading infection I do not advise lubrication of the tube with any jelly, but spray the trachea with a 4% local anaesthesia with, for example, the Mackintosh spray, before intubation. This is a very useful technique, especially when the patient breathes spontaneously after intubation. The tube is a foreign body and is better tolerated if the mucosa is anaesthetised. This will also help to reduce the amount of anaesthetic used.

5.2.5 Nasal Intubation

The nasal tube has to be well lubricated and passed gently through the most suitable nostril until it reaches the pharynx. The larynx is exposed as for oral intubation and with the help of a Magill's forceps the tube is lifted into the larynx and gently pushed down.

5.2.6 Oral Intubation under Local Anaesthesia with a Sedated Patient

Spray 4% local anaesthesia on the tongue and pharynx. Once the area is insensitive, the epiglottis can be exposed with a curved laryngoscope which is bladed and also sprayed. After a few minutes it can be lifted up, the cord and trachea sprayed, and the tube induced. This method can easily be carried out on a well-sedated patient (bronchography).

5.2.7 Difficulties and Complications ·

5.2.7.1 Anatomical Problems

The patient cannot open his mouth wide enough or has extensive tumours in the mouth. This should certainly be checked before operation at the pre-anaesthetic examination and ruled out. It may possibly be necessary to perform blind nasal intubation with spontaneous respiration. The patient might have short and fat neck together with the so-called horse tooth. Be sure to give sufficient relaxants and use an inducer or mandrill. (Mandrills are only used to increase the curve of the tube and as a guide to where the tube can be pushed over.)

5.2.7.2 Insufficient Relaxation

Firstly it is difficult to expose the larynx clearly and secondly at the attempt of intubation a laryngeal spasm may occur. Induce enough relaxation and wait for its full effect. *Never use force for intubation.* Forceful intubation can lead to injuries of the epiglottis and to post-operative respiratory complications.

5.2.7.3 Complications

Complications in intubation appear mainly when the lumen of the tube is obstructed or misplaced (see Fig. 5.10).

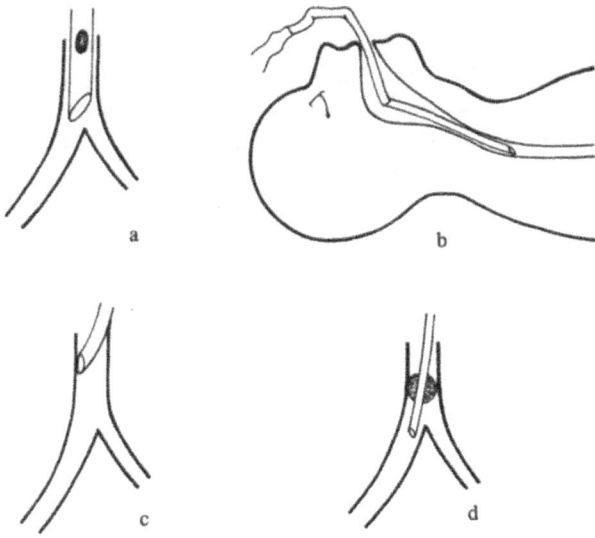

Fig. 5.10. *a* blocked lumen, *b* kinked tube, *c* bevel against trachea. Air goes in but does not go out, *d* tube lies in one bronchus (check both lungs), *e* tube slides out (fix it properly), *f* tube is in the oesophagus (common). The bag does not in flate properly and the patient can sometimes phonate.

a) Infections and oedema of the trachea and epiglottis are caused by unsterile and wrong technique; antibiotics and cortisones are the answer.

b) Hoarseness and a sore throat can occur when the intubation was rather traumatic, but it disappears quickly.

Remember: intubation is not a surgical procedure. It is a technique which can be learned and which helps to keep the patient alive during anaesthesia.

5.3 Artificial Ventilation of the Lungs

Intermittant Positive Pressure Respiration can be either controlled or assisted respiration.

5.3.1 Controlled Respiration

In controlled respiration the respiratory muscles are paralysed and the lungs are artificially inflated with a breathing bag. The normal respiration is altered and the physiology reversed. Instead of air being sucked into the lungs, air is forced into it by positive pressure. The venous return to the heart which is assisted under normal inspiration is partly prevented by the rise of intrathoracic pressure. The alveolar capillaries are compressed by the inspiration, limiting the blood flow and the gas exchange. In this way I.P.P.R. partly influences the circulation. This effect can be minimised by a short inspiratory time and a longer expiratory time, in the relation of one to three. A normally fit patient can easily compensate this negative effect; however, if there is already a considerable reduction of circulation (R-sied H.F.), I.P.P.R. without a negative phase can cause a remarkable affect.

5.3.2 Assisted Respiration

In assisted respiration the patient is partially paralysed, and breathing but inadequately. The breathing bag is squeezed in time with the patient's inspiration and therefore the respiratory volume is increased (see Chap. 1).

To be most physiological, artificial ventilation should be according to the age and the lung compliance of the patient. By lung compliance we understand the elasticity of the lungs, which means pressure: cm H_2O used per litre volume. The normal compliance for an adult is 0.1 litre/cm H_2O. The pressure used for inflating the lungs, however, should be kept as low as possible and not be above 15-20 cm H_2O. Pressure above 30 cm H_2O results in an interruption of the venosity of pulmonary flow (see Fig. 5.11). Pressure above 40 cm H_2O would result in a complete standstill of the alveolar capillary flow and therefore no possibility of diffusion, together with increased pressure to the right side of the heart. These negative haemodynamic effects can be *partly* compensated by using intermittant and positive-negative pressure respiration. By prolonging the expiratory period in a relation of one to two, the so-called middle pressure can be lowered (see Fig. 5.12).

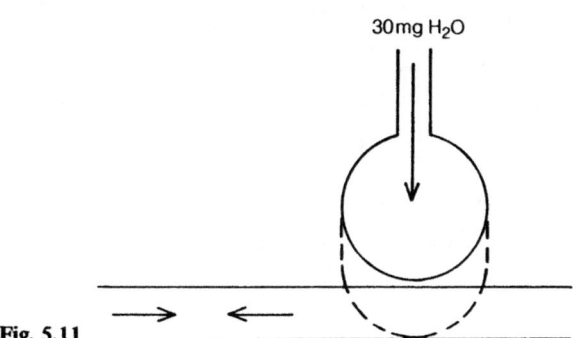

30mg H_2O

Fig. 5.11

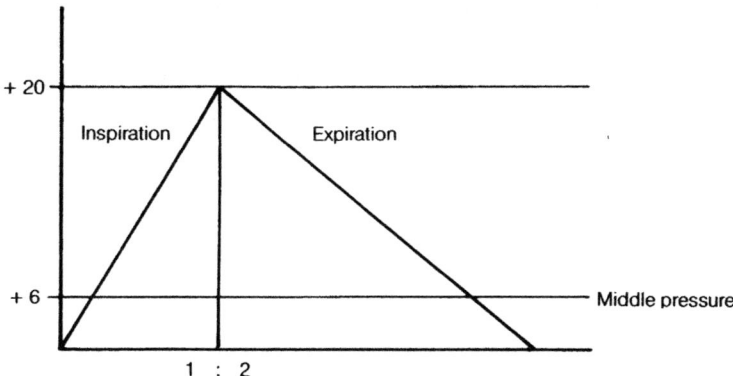

Fig. 5.12

+ 20

Inspiration

Expiration

+ 6

Middle pressure

1 : 2

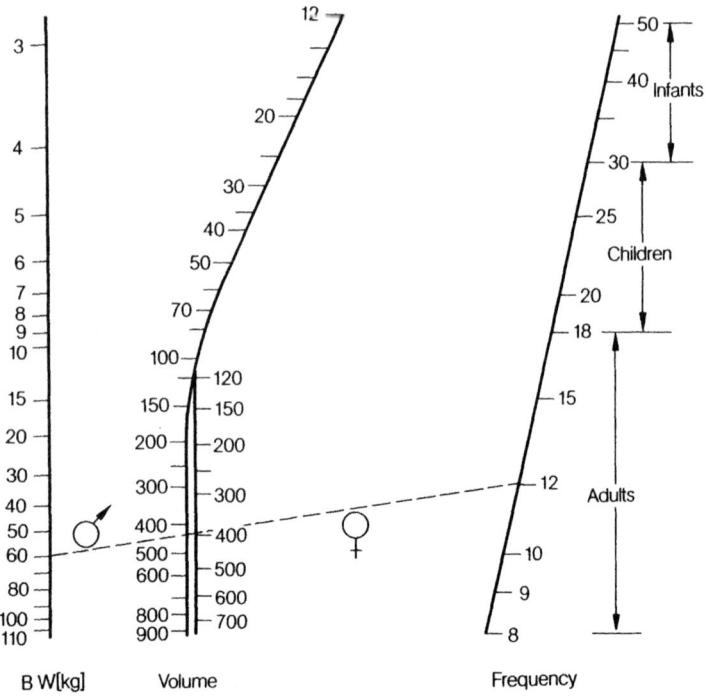

Fig. 5.13. Draw a line between B W and frequency (age) – the line will indicate the volume, (from Stöcker, Narkose. Georg Thieme Verlag Stuttgart, 4th ed., 1976)

Other important factors are the *frequency* and the *volume* of the artificial ventilation. If it is too frequent the volume is reduced, the dead-space ventilation is increased and no time is left for the diffusion. According to Roughton at least 0.3 s are needed for a normal diffusion. On the other hand, due to the haemodynamic effect, the inspiration should not be kept too long. Observation of your *own* ventilation is possibly a good guide (see Fig. 5.13).

Chapter 6

Anaesthesia Techniques and Equipment

General anaesthesia can be achieved by:

 a) Intravenous anaesthesia, e.g. Ketalar
 b) Inhalation anaesthesia, e.g. halothane, ether
 c) Combination anaesthesia, e.g. IV induction and inhalation anaesthesia

The most common method is combination anaesthesia, using a powerful IV hypnotic, e.g. barbiturates, for inducing sleep, while anaesthesia is maintained with inhalation anaesthesia and muscle relaxants. Inhalation anaesthesia can be divided into four groups:

 1) Open method
 2) Half-open method
 3) Half-closed method
 4) Closed method

The main differences in the techniques are (1) the existence of a reservoir, which means the possibility of artificial ventilation (2) and rebreathing or not rebreathing of the expiratory air, which means a possibility of absorbing CO_2 (see Table 6.1).

Table 6.1

Method	Reservoir	Rebreathing of expiratory air
(1)	−	−
(2)	+	−
(3)	+	+
(4)	+	+

6.1 Open Method (see Fig. 6.1)

There is a free passage of atmospheric air enriched with anaesthetic gas or vapour. There is no control over the inspiratory or expiratory amount of air and no resource for active ventilation.

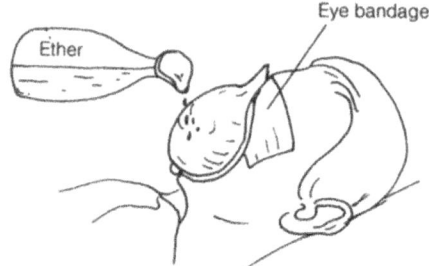

Fig. 6.1

6.2 Half-Open Method or Semi-Open System

The anaesthetic gas is given through a tube system via a reservoir to the patient. The expiration air disappears over a non-rebreathing valve, e.g. Ruben valve, into the atmospheric air. The presence of an air reservoir presents the option of artificial ventilation. The available equipment includes the Ruben, Epstein – Mackintosh – Oxford = E.M.O. – and the "Afya" (Draeger) anaesthesia machines.

The E.M.O. and "Afya" anaesthesia machines and their techniques are the most logical, reliable and simplest methods of administering anaesthesia. The simplicity of these machines accounts for their safety. With the apparatus atmospheric air can be saturated with exact doses of ether and with a small addition of halothane. There are also reliable means of inflating the patient's lungs, using the Oxford Inflating Bellow in conjuction with the E.M.O. machine (see Fig. 6.2) or the Inflating Bellow of the "Afya" machine (see Fig. 6.14).

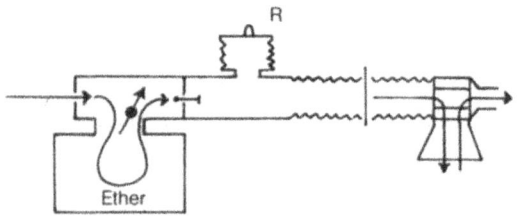

Fig. 6.2. Schematic diagram of half-open system

The "AFYA" Anaesthesia Machine

("AFYA" comes from Kiswahili national Language in Tanzania and it means "HEALTH").

From our many years of experience with the half-open anaesthesia technique at the Machame Lutheran Hospital in Tanzania, the "AFYA" Anaesthetic machine has been developed and built by the Drägerwerk, AG Lübeck — West Germany.

The system is based on the "draw-over" method and can be used for r control and spontaneous ventilation.

The range of technical modification or assembling possibilities range from the simple portable unit (combination A and B) until the setting up of an anaesthetic machine with the possibility of adding additional oxygen, control of end-inspiratory pressure as well as respirometry (combination E). In this case the simple half-open anaesthetic system offers a maximum of optical controls.

The main item is an ether vapouriser with one valve, together with two elephant or rubber tubes, a breathing bag and expiratory valve.

For paediatric anaesthesia the tubes, valve, and bag should be changed to a smaller size.

The system has practically no dead space and low respiratory resistant. For paediatric anaesthesia we consider it suitable. Advantages of this anaesthetic machine:

— safe anaesthetic technique.
— Low cost in running, no compressed cases are needed, one bottle ether, offers many anaesthesias.
— minimum dead space
— low resistance
— possibility of adding all necessary optic controls.
   a) Respirometry
   b) Pressure control of insuflating pressure.
— possibility of giving up to 100% oxygen
— suitable for paediatric anaesthesia
— easy to transport
— easy to clean.

The other addition is a non-rebreathing valve at the end of the elephant tubing or connection to the patient. In this way a simple non-return system is provided whether the patient respiration is spontaneous or controlled.

6.2.1 The Choice of Ether

Unfortunately ether has an evil reputation as far as toxity is concerned, which is largely attributable to the fact that ether has been given in too large amounts and in inaccurate dosages. All anaesthetic agents are toxic when used to produce deep anaesthesia. Ether has been used for a long time to produce deep anaesthesia and it is unreasonable that the bad reputation of ether in this respect should be allowed to persist (J. Parkhause, etc.). When a muscle relaxant is used for anaesthesia and the quantities of the general anaesthetic ether can be kept accordingly to a minimum, i.e. to produce amnesia only, ether is probably one of the safest general anaesthetics. In fact, if 2%-4% ether vapour is administered to the patient, he will be awake and talking after the end of the operation, just as if he had been given nitrous oxide or halothane.

Post operation vomiting under these conditions is as rare as under nitrous oxide and halothane.

6.2.2 The Choice of Air

Atmospheric air is cheap, is humidified and provides adequate O_2. With liquid anaesthetic ether the quantity of vapour required for the maintenance of light anaesthesia makes only an insignificant difference to the percentage of oxygen in the inspired air, and an unconscious patient immobile on the operation table can be fully oxygenated with this mixture. *Anoxia is usually due to inadequate ventilation.* The result is either respiratory depression or respiratory obstruction and is consequently associated with carbon dioxide retention. Often the problem is not exclusively one of anoxia, but of carbon-dioxide retention. Therefore the answer is not so much an addition of oxygen, as the *institution of adequate ventilation.* I do not want to imply that there are no circumstances under which oxygen should be added, but recent study (Nandrup) reveals that adequate ventilation with light ether and room air results in oxygen saturation equal to, or higher than, normal. Furthermore, atmospheric air is already humidified to such a degree that prolonged administration is possible, even though a non-return system, without fear of detriment to the patients lungs.

6.2.3 The Choice of the Non-Return System

Considering the number of errors the rebreathing system implies, the non-rebreathing system is certainly better where cheap anaesthetic gases (air/ether) are used for anaesthesia. The technique is simple and the anaesthetist does not depend on the proper use of soda lime and elaborate apparatus. The patient is assured of a fresh supply of gases with each inspiration and the composition of the inspired gas mixture is accurately known. Hygiene is an important factor. The only parts of the apparatus through which the patient can rebreathe are the endotracheal tube and the valve. They must both be sterilised between cases. As an "optional extra" the expiratory side of the valve can be connected with a respiratory volumeter to control the respiratory volume of the patient. I am convinced that the correct administration of ether as an anaesthetic agent in air through a non-return system is a logical, safe and economic method of anaesthesia, even today.

6.3 Half-Closed System

Anaesthetic gas which originates from a gas cylinder (compressed gas) is given through a tube system. Only part of the expired air disappears, the rest goes back to the patient via a CO_2 absorber and an air reservoir. Together with fresh gas from the machine, the gas goes back to the patient via a valve system (see Fig. 6.3). The technique provides the possibility of different anaesthetic methods, but it should be kept in mind that there is also the danger of more errors by technical failure.

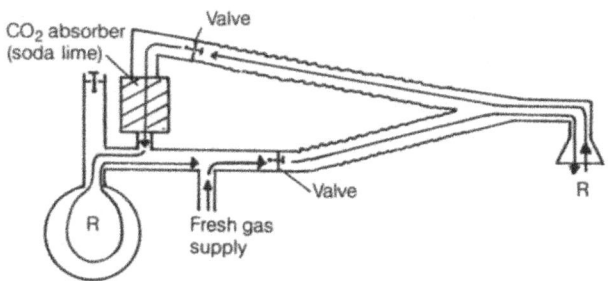

Fig. 6.3. Schematic diagram of half-closed system

6.4 Closed System

This method allows complete rebreathing of the expired air and CO_2 and elimination through an absorber and an air reservoir or breathing bag. Only the necessary metabolic O_2 is added.

Other technical equipment absolutely necessary for anaesthesia are: instruments for maintenance of airway and the items for performing intubation (see Figs. 6.4-6.13).

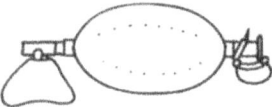

Face mask

Fig. 6.4. Double-ended self-inflating bag

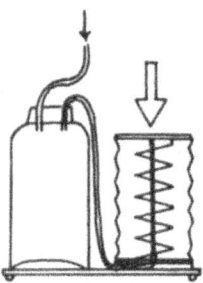

Fig. 6.5. Foot-operated section pump

6.5 PEEP Respiration

Definition: PEEP = positive end expiratory pressure, positive pressure of respiration in the end expiratory phase.

The pressure course in the expiratory phase can be influenced with modern respirator equipment. The mean *respiratory position* and thus the main intrathoracic pressure can be lowered compared to the zero position by setting negative values or raised by setting positive values.

In the setting of the positive values (PEEP, CPPV), an expiration pressure of up to +20 cm of water is possible.

Note: A fundamental distinction must be made between non-damaged and disturbed pulmonary function in the adjustment of the respirator.

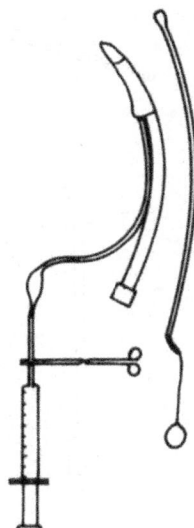

Fig. 6.6. Different size Magill or Oxford tubes with connector and inflating syringe and Plastic-Stilette

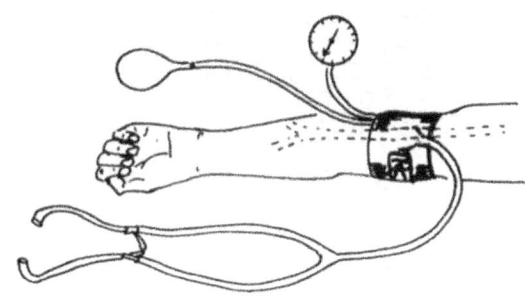

Fig. 6.7. Stethoscope and B P machine

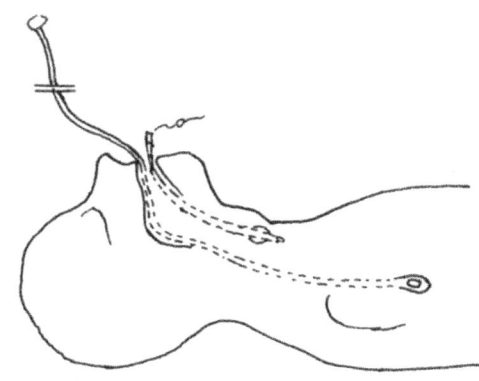

Fig. 6.8. Oesophagus-Stethoscope

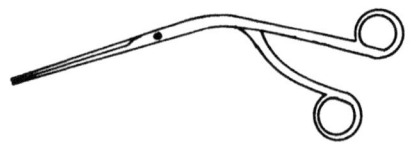

Fig. 6.9. Magill introducing forceps

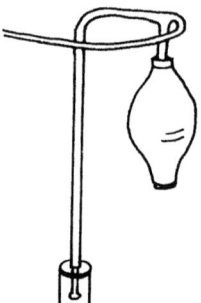

Fig. 6.10. Spray (endotracheal)

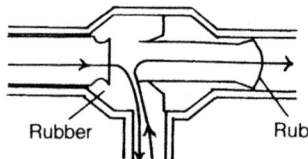

Rubber   Rubber   **Fig. 6.11.** Ambu valve (rubber)

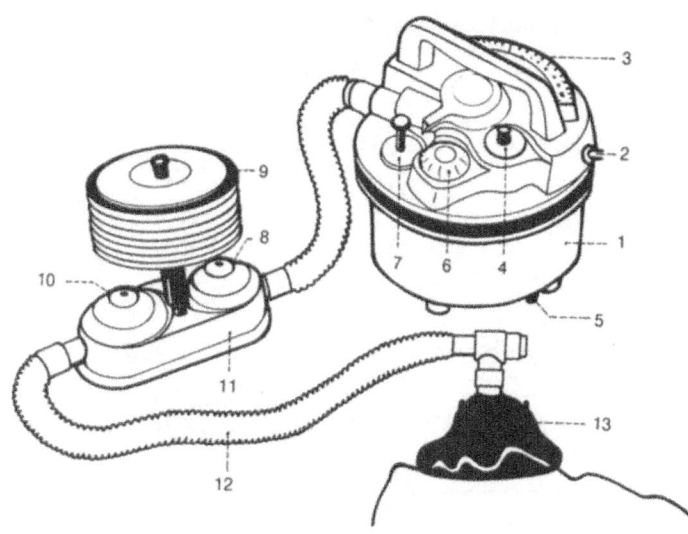

Fig. 6.12. *1* E.M.O. Inhaler, *2* air inlet to E.M.O. (must remain unobstructed at all times), *3* concentration control (1-20% Val.) *4* temperature compensator indicator, the black band must show; if the red band is visible the apparatus is too hot refill water at −, *5* water filler (for water jacket), *6* ether filler knob (only fill when concent. is open), *7* ether level indicator, *8* unidirectional valve inlet to O.I.B., *9* Oxford Inflating Bellows, *10* unidirectional valve outlet − must be removed (Magnet) when a non-re-breathing valve (13) is used, *11* O.I.B. Unit, *12* breathing tubing, *13* non-re-breathing valve

The interplay of the following variables of adjustable parameters is decisive for the effect on respiration:

1. Frequency of respiration (f)
2. Volume of respiration (V_T)
3. Respiration pressure over the airways (AP)
4. Quotient of respiration time
5. The flow of inspiration and expiration
6. PEEP

Effects of PEEP

Application of PEEP leads to a marked improvement of pulmonary function. It is at present the best possible type of therapy for influencing pulmonary gas exchange in the clinical course of acute respiratory disturbances. However, this form of respiration therapy frequently also leads to an impairment of

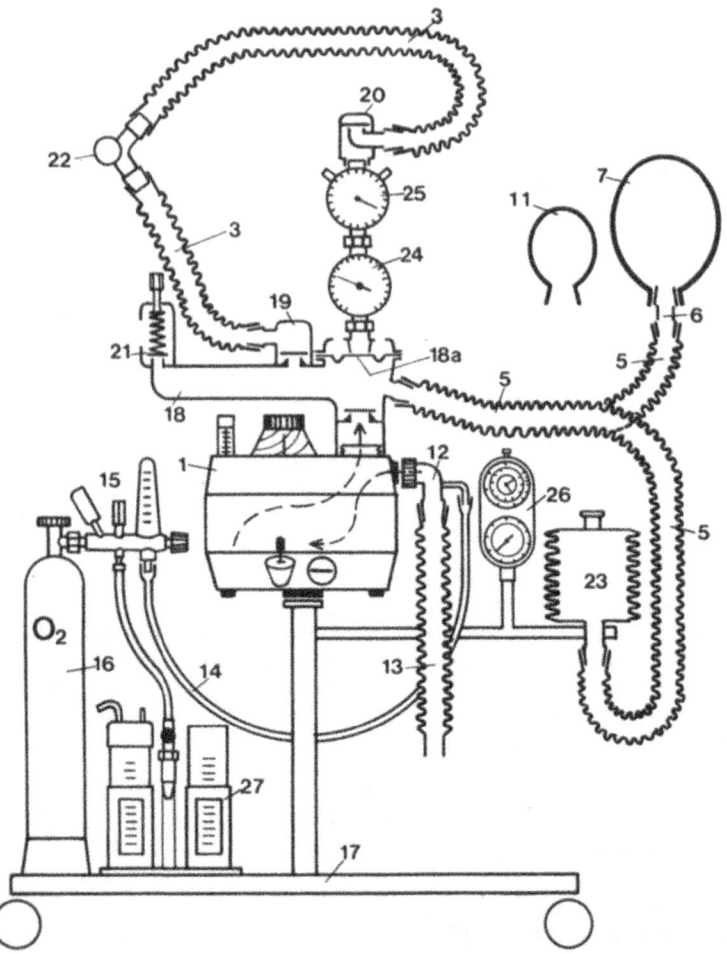

Fig. 6.13. Combination "E": complete equipment combination with all "modules" for hospital (stationary) use. *1* CATO; *2* ether vaporizer; *3* Corrugated tubes 1 m long 22 dia; *5* Corrugated tube 1 m long 22 dia; *6* Connection port for respiratory bag; *7* Respiratory bag, large; *11* Respiratory bag, small; *12* O_2 connection piece; *13* O_2 reservoir tube; *14* O_2 connection tube; *15* O_2 pressure reducer with flowmeter; *16* O_2 cylinder; *17* Trolley; *18* Valve chamber with; *18a* Expiratory control valve; *19* Inspiratory valve; *20* Expiratory valve; *21* Relief valve; *22* Y-piece; *23* Respiratory bellows; *24* Respiratory pressure gauge; *25* Minute Volumeter; *26* Anaesthesia timer/sphygmomanometer; *27* Bronchial aspirator; *28* Connecting arm for item 26

cardiovascular function. Several factors are responsible for the alterations in the cardiac output and organ blood flow under PEEP respiration.

The pulmonary capillary pressure normally correlates well with the mean left atrial pressure and the left ventricular filling pressure.

Exceptions are elevations of the pulmonary vascular resistance, mitral stenosis, tachycardia, etc.

Note: It is not the absolute mean left atrial pressure (in relation to the atmospheric pressure) which is the actual determinant for left ventricular filling, but the transmural pressure which is equal to the intrapleural pressure. This rises with increasing PEEP in a non-predictable fashion.

PEEP leads to an elevation of functional residual capacity, and thus to a shift in the ratio of FRC to the *Verschlußvolumen* (closing volume) in favor of FRC. Each 5 cm H_2O elevation of PEEP leads to an increase of FRC by around 400-500 ml.

One refers to the optimum or best PEEP when the cardiac output as well as the total compliance is highest and the quotient dead space/inspiratory volume are lowest. The best PEEP is normally in a range up to 15 cm water and depends on the FRC of the patient before ventilation.

Increasing PEEP increases the static compliance, but worsens the dynamic compliance in end-expiratory pressure of more than 10 cm H_2O. The quotient dead space/inspiratory volume increases. PAO and intrapulmonary pressure respectively increase *and* decrease under PEEP.

The two parameters are not a good measure for evaluating a best PEEP, since they also increase or decrease after the critical PEEP limit has been exceeded. Cardiac output and O_2 fall immediately after the critical PEEP has been exceeded.

Dead space/inspiratory volume increase even with optimal volume substitution.

a) The raised intrathoracic pressure brings about a reduction of venous return to the heart. This results in a reduction of the filling pressures in the right side of the heart and thus to a lowering of the stroke volume of the right side of the heart.
b) An increase in the vascular resistance in the pulmonary circulation is observed in severe respiratory distress syndromes. This can lead to dilatation of the right ventricle and a displacement of the septum into the left ventricle.
c) The stroke volume of the left ventricle is likewise lowered. A deterioration of the contractility plays an additional role in the reduced filling.
d) Kidney function can deteriorate in consequence of the altered cardiac function. In addition, a redistribution of intrarenal perfusion by PEEP as well as venous congestion may play a role here. An increased secretion of antidiuretic hormone during respiration with PEEP can also promote retention of water.

e) The liver function is influenced by PEEP under respiration by the impediment to venous return into the thorax as well as a reduction of portal vein perfusion and biliary drainage.

Since a precise analysis of pulmonary and circulatory function can only be performed in the most well equipped intensive care wards, one must resort to simpler measurements which permit the optimal pulmonary function and oxygen transport to be estimated for adapting the respiration pattern of each individual patient.

Parameters which are simple to determine are the total static compliance and the mixed venous partial pressure of oxygen. They permit an adaption of the respiration form of PEEP in order to achieve an optimal oxygen transport in the patient:

1. The total static compliance of the respiratory system provides an indicator for the range of the best extensibility and thus the ideal respiration in terms of lung mechanics.
2. The partial pressure of oxygen in the mixed venous blood is the result of three factors: pulmonary gas exchange, oxygen transport due to the cardiac output, and peripheral oxygen consumption.

If the PEEP has to be raised beyond the normal values, e.g. in very severely restricted pulmonary gas exchange, this mostly results in lowering of cardiac output. To limit and treat the cardiovascular side-effects of machine respiration with PEEP, three methods are available:

1. Individual adaptation of the respiration pattern to the patients
2. A therapeutic expansion of the circulating blood volume
3. A pharmacological treatment of circulatory depression, e.g. with dopamine

Indications for PEEP (CPPV)

1. Impossibility of achieving an alveolar partial pressure of oxygen greater than 70 mmHg at an oxygen concentration of 0.5 in the inspiratory gas mixture with IPPV (= Intermittent Positive Pressure Ventilation).
2. The alveolar arterial oxygen difference is greater than 300 in IPPB with an FIO 2 = 1.0.
3. Impossibility of shunt reduction during IPPB (despite carrying out all conventional therapeutic and prophylactic measures: cardiac therapy, prevention or correction of a fluid overloading, changing position, prophylaxis of atelectasia, therapy of pneumonia, bronchial cleansing, etc.).

66

4. A functional residual capacity (FRC) less than 50% of the normal value
5. Pulmonary oedema
6. Ventilation of patients who have almost drowned
7. Withdrawal from the respirator
    a) IMV= Intermittent Mandatory Ventilation or Intermittent Dement
       Ventilation with PEEP
    b) Spontaneous respiration with PEEP

Contraindications for PEEP (CPPV)

1. Manifest or latent dextrocardiac insufficiency
2. Uncorrected hypovolemia
3. Hypotension
4. Fall in PAO_2 despite proper adjustment of the respirator with the occurrence of raised shunting due to redistribution of the blood in non-ventilated alveoli (elevation of the mean airway pressure and the pulmonary volume). Overinflation of normal alveoli (especially in patients with chronic obstructive pulmonary disease) can lead to an increase in the dead space/inspiratory volume, and thus to a fall in the PAO_2 with a rise of $PACO_2$.

Summary

The positive end-expiratory pressure (PEEP) influences the pulmonary capillary wall pressure (PCWP) in two ways:

1. Elevation of the intrapleural pressure
2. Elevation of the pulmonary vascular resistance by pressure transmission.

Chapter 7

General Anaesthesia Techniques

It is the intention of these notes on anaesthesia to demonstrate safe, simple and effective anaesthesia methods, mainly used in developing countries, or in disaster situations, where anaesthesia is performed by medical assistants or auxiliaries. Therefore much emphasis is put on the demonstration of the half-open, the half-closed and other cheap and simple anaesthetic methods. Usually anaesthesia is performed by the combination anaesthesia technique using an IV anaesthetic agent for a quick induction and maintenance of anaesthesia with an inhalation agent. Anaesthesia without intubation (no ideal method).

7.1 Barbiturate — Ether — Air

Premedicate, carefully prepare all anaesthesia equipment, and set up an IV drip. Give 3 mg barbiturate/kg body wt. (for example: thiopentone) IV. After the patient has lost consciousness, air or possibly air and O_2 is inhaled via a non-breathing valve and well-fitting mask. Increase the ether concentration after every fifth breath by 1% up to 10%-15%. Maintain this concentration until the surgical stage of anaesthesia is achieved in about 10-15 min. As soon as the patient tolerates surgical manoeuvres, reduce the ether concentration to 8%-6% volume ether to maintain anaesthesia. If a halothane-vaporiser is available, the induction period can be reduced. Fill the vaporiser with 5 ml halothane. Set the concentration on 1% and start induction as before. As soon as the surgical stage is reached, discontinue halothane and maintain anaesthesia with ether. Complications often appear during the induction period, especially with barbiturates. Commonly there is a period of apnea, holding breath, coughing, vomiting or laryngospasm. The reasons are either too fast an application or barbiturates or the irritating effect of ether. In all these cases, it might be necessary to stop anaesthesia, clear and support the airway and maybe assist respiration with O_2, until the patient is settled. Then start anaesthesia again.

Always be sure that there is a free airway! There may also be a sudden fall of B P and pulse rate with impaired circulation which requires an increase of infusion therapy and reduction of anaesthesia (see Fig. 7.1). During the induction period the use of a small dose of barbiturates, followed by halothane air, is usually smoother and less traumatic. The time of induction can also be reduced.

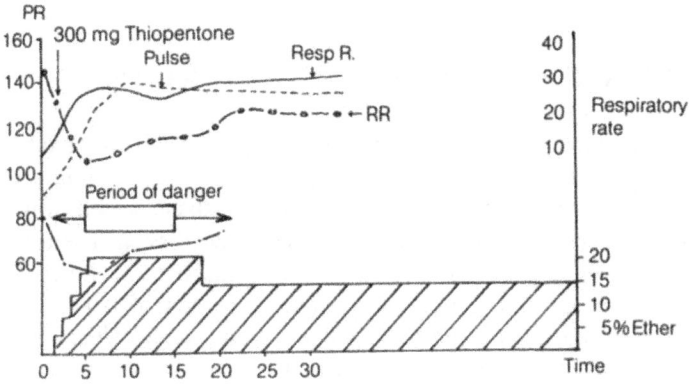

Fig. 7.1

7.2 Ketalar — Ether — Air

Ketalar can be used for IV or IM induction of anaesthesia. The IM use of Ketalar for induction is very useful in paediatric anaesthesia: 1-2 mg Ketalar/kg body wt. IV or 5 mg Ketalar/kg body wt. IM. As soon as the patient loses consciousness, continue with a well-fitting non-rebreathing valve and mask and increase the ether concentration up to 10%. The duration of Ketalar is usually enough to reach the surgical stage of anaesthesia with ether. The severe saliva production caused by Ketalar and ether make premedication with atropine essential and even frequent sucking necessary. B P and pulse rate are often increased by this technique.

7.3 Neuroleptica — Ether — Air

To avoid the dangerous and often traumatic induction period associated with barbiturates the use of neuroleptica has been widely practised for premedication, followed by ether air.

Premedication: 0.3 mg dehydrobenzperidol/kg body wt. or 0.1 mg halo-peridol/kg body wt. +0.2 mg Diazepam/kg body wt. 1 h before operation.

Fill the halothane-vaporiser with 5 ml halothane and set at 1%. Induce anaesthesia with a non-rebreathing valve, a mask and halothane air (1%). As soon as the patient loses consciousness start to raise the ether concentration by 2% and increase after every fifth breath by 1% up to 10%-15%. Halothane is then discontinued.

7.4 Induction Followed by O_2+N_2O+Halothane

This technique is usually used in the half-open or half-closed inhalation method. O_2+N_2O+halothane make a good hypnotic and analgetic mixture with poor relaxation, unless a high concentration of halothane is used, which, however, causes severe respiratory and cardio-vascular depression. The technique is pre-ferably used in combination with a muscle relaxant and will be discussed in the next chapter. In the half-open method the flow of gases has to be kept very high: about three times the patient's respiratory volume, which makes anaesthesia quite expensive. Take care that the concentration of O_2 is at least 25% of the patient's respiratory volume, on average 1 O_2: 2 N_2O. 0.8%-1.5% halothane or 6%-8% ether.

7.5 Maintenance of Anaesthesia

Anaesthesia must be maintained at a point where the patient tolerates surgical practice, combined with adequate muscle relaxation. After the start of the operation when the patient is well settled, the saturation of anaesthetic gas is sufficient and the dosage can be reduced to the maintenance level. It is a com-mon mistake to go too low with the ether concentration, which results in the waking up of the patient. For a normally fit patient, concentration of 5%-6% ether is necessary to maintain anaesthesia and good muscle relaxation without the addition of muscle relaxants.

7.6 Monitoring

7.6.1 Respiration

Special attention has to be given to the maintenance of the airway from the very beginning of anaesthesia (see Chap. 9). As soon as the patient loses consciousness a clean airway has to be observed — sometimes by supporting the jaw or installing an airway. Respiration is usually well maintained during a normal dosage of ether anaesthesia. There will be an extra deep breath every 2-3 min, which is physiologically normal. The respiration should otherwise be regular and of adequate depth. Deep breaths, however, can occur in deep anaesthesia and should not be taken as a sign of light anaesthesia. Seesaw respiration (tracheal tug), are alarming indications of insufficient respiration and the beginning of catastrophy. Stop anaesthesia, clear the airway and maintain adequate ventilation, even assisting respiration until the patient is settled again.

While controlling respiration, control the fresh gas supply, estimate ventilation and be sure that the air reaches the alveoli. Watch for leaks, blocked valves and whether the thorax expands. Finally, the finger nails, the mucous membranes and the blood from the surgical field should indicate a good O_2 tension.

7.6.2 Circulation

It is characteristic of ether anaesthesia that cardiac output and arterial pressure are well maintained. However, in elderly or in drug-taking patients (especially when sympathetic-blocking and sedative drugs are taken) this does not always apply. It also depends on an adequate fluid replacement during the operation (see Chap. 12). Ectopic heartbeats are common under ether anaesthesia and probably an expression of increased sympathetic activity. They might be accompanied by a fall of cardiac output. If there is adequate O_2 tension in the blood, no action or treatment are necessary.

Halothane inhalation anaesthesia with spontaneous respiration is often associated with a fall of BP and bradycardia (see Fig. 7.2), which has to be carefully observed and controlled by reducing halothane, even giving atropine and more infusion. Halothane inhalation anaesthesia under spontaneous respiration is, however, not ideal.

7.6.3 O_2 Substitute

Atmospheric air is adequate in light surgical ether air anaesthesia in a normally fit and healthy patient. The following conditions, however, require additional 1-2 litres O_2/min:

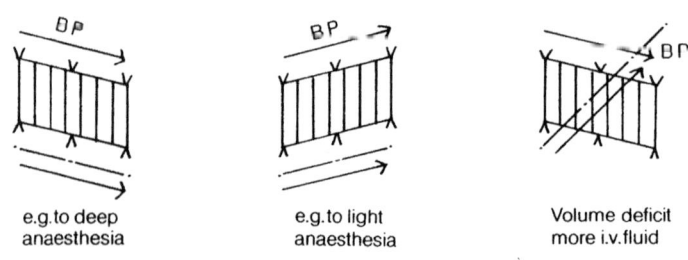

e.g. to deep anaesthesia   e.g. to light anaesthesia   Volume deficit more i.v. fluid

Fig. 7.2. Typical move of B P and pulse

a) Acute and chronic chest diseases
b) Acute and chronic heart diseases
c) Low Hgb. (under 10 g%)
d) Trendelenburg or Lithotomic position
e) Heavy premedication

Under normal circumastances a patient breathing ether air will have an O_2 saturation above 90% but if respiration is depressed, e.g. with an abdominal tumour or after heavy premedication, the saturation will fall so that O_2 substitute is necessary. The effects of O_2 *starvation* include prolonged recovery, restlessness, progressive C.C.F., bradycardia and sudden cardiac arrest (see Fig. 7.3).

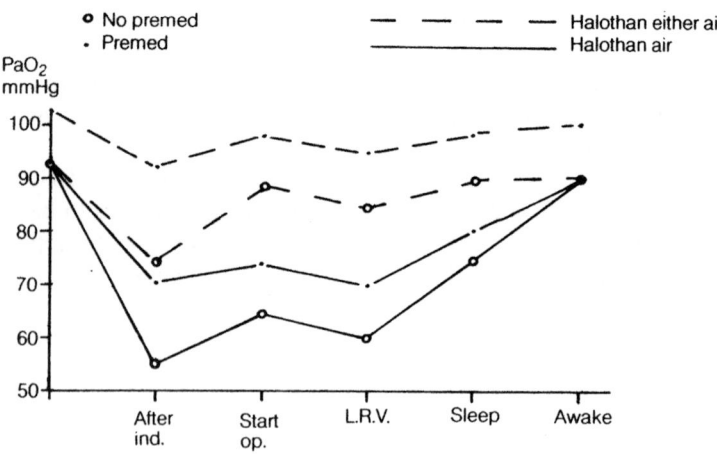

Fig. 7.3. Arterial oxygen tensions during anaesthesia with ether and halothane

7.7 Recovery

Average anaesthesia can be stopped 5-10 min before the end of the operation. Ether can be stopped even earlier and anaesthesia continued with halothane, which loses effect faster. *Remember: Never let a patient out of your hands before you are sure that the respiration and circulation are well maintained.*

7.8 Relaxation and Artificial Ventilation

The great advantage of the muscle relaxants are that the general anaesthetic drugs are used only to produce a *slight anaesthesia* or better, *amnesia*, which means a short recovery period. Relaxation is achieved by administering a muscle relaxation drug (see Fig. 7.4).

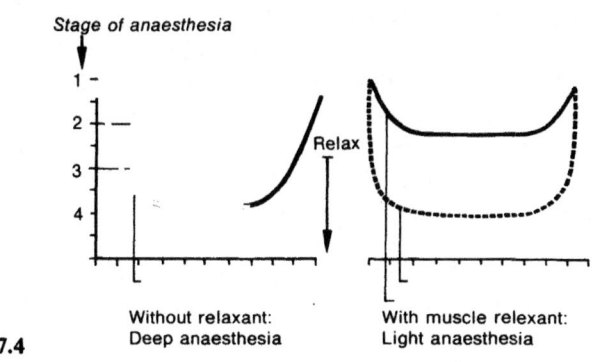

Fig. 7.4

Fig. 7.4

The relaxant, however, also relaxes the respiratory muscles, so that these drugs can only be used when the anaesthetist is adequately able to take over the ventilation of the patient. This means, the anaesthetist must be able to intubate and perform positive pressure ventilation, which requires a minimum knowledge of the physiology of the respiratory system and the necessary equipment. I personally want to emphasise that every medical auxilliary who is asked to perform anaesthesia should *make an effort to set up the technical equipment necessary for intubation and learn to intubate.*
Intubation makes anaesthesia safer and easier.

7.8.1 Technique

Premedicate (see Chap. 4) and ascertain that all necessary technical equipment is there and in working condition (see Chap. 5).

Induce anaesthesia with an induction agent such as one of the following:

Thiopentone	3-5 mg/kg body wt.	i.v.
Ketalar	2 mg/kg body wt.	i.v.
Epontol	5 mg/kg body wt.	i.v.
Halothane − Air − O_2		

After induction and amnesia of the patient, give a short-acting muscle relaxant, e.g. 1 mg Scoline/kg body wt. IV. Assist respiration and after full relaxation is achieved control ventilation with O_2 enriched air using a bellow, valve and mask. If there is no possibility of O_2 substitution let the patient breathe deeply before and during the induction period. This will increase the O_2 tension and partly cover the time of apnea during intubation. As soon as there is complete relaxation, endotracheal intubation is performed as explained in Chap. 8. This can be performed easily and atraumatically during the short period of relaxation. A relaxed patient does not cough and a laryngospasm is unlikely. After intubation, connect with the anaesthesia machine or another source of artificial ventilation and continue controlled ventilation. Ether concentration is set on 8%-15% *if anaesthesia is to continue under spontaneous respiration.* Usually by the time the spontaneous respiration returns, the patient will breathe quietly and is ready for surgery. Ether concentration can then be reduced to a maintenance level of 6%-8%.

There is a tendency to hyperventilate the patient during the period of controlled ventilation. Ventilation should be adequate. Hyperventilation will avoid or prolong spontaneous respiration. Hypoventilation will, however, usually lead to more serious complications.

If relaxation is maintained by the use of a muscle relaxant, which is *the ideal method*, ether, (or whatever is used as the inhalation anaesthetic) is required only to achieve *hypnosis* or *amnesia.*

After induction and intubation, set ether concentration at 6% volume, ventilate and as soon as the neuromuscular function returns, maintain relaxation by giving preferably long-acting muscle relaxants, e.g. 0.2 mg curarine/kg body wt. or 2 mg gallamine/kg body wt. or 0.02 mg Pavolon/kg body wt. or a Scoline drip.

After the start of the operation and the patient is well settled, i.e. easy to ventilate and showing no signs of awareness, the ether concentration can be reduced 3%-5% to *maintain amnesia.* If relaxation is inadequate give a repeat dosage of one-third of the initial dose of the muscle relaxant.

7.8.2 Maintenance

By the use of a relaxant, the normal lung physiology is interrupted and the ventilation of the lungs has to be taken over by the anaesthetist as physiologically as possible. All the main body functions must also be constantly monitored (see Figs. 7.5, 7.6 and 7.7). Both hyper- and hypoventilation should be avoided. The use of an oesophagus-stethoscope controls the pulse rate and respiration. Bear in mind that every patient loses 500 ml fluid per hour with an open abdomen (see Chap. 2).

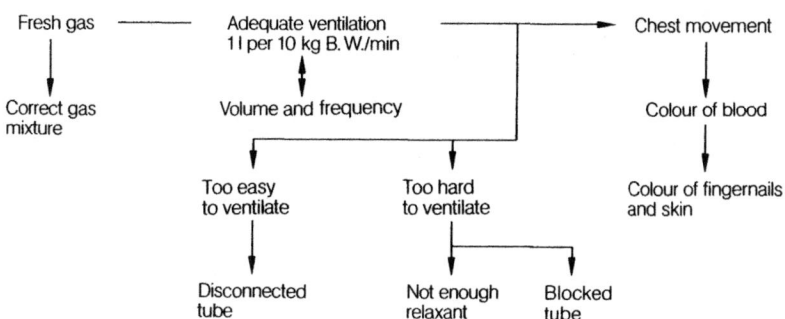

Fig. 7.5

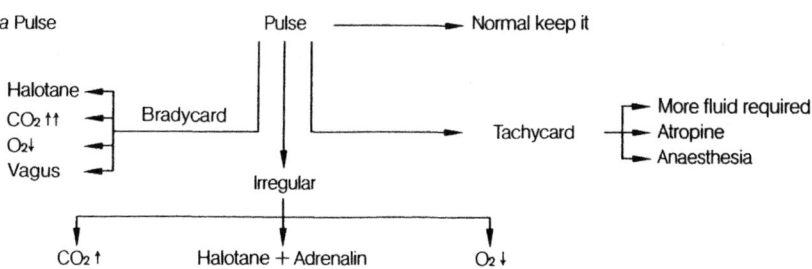

Fig. 7.6. *a* Pulse

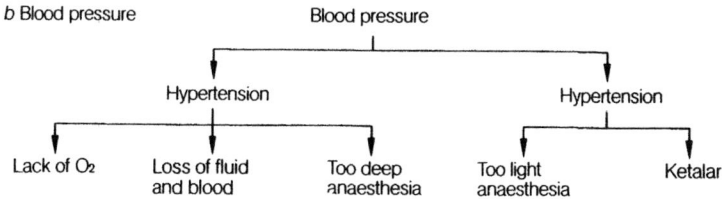

Fig. 7.6. *b* Blood pressure

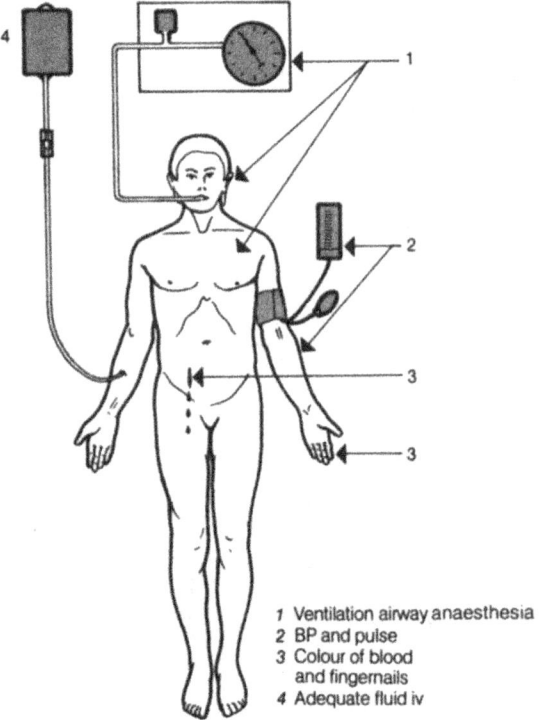

1 Ventilation airway anaesthesia
2 BP and pulse
3 Colour of blood
  and fingernails
4 Adequate fluid iv

Fig. 7.7

7.8.3 Recovery Period

To avoid an unduly long recovery period after ether anaesthesia switch off
the ether vaporiser 5-10 min before the end of the operation. If necessary,
anaesthesia can be continued with a small dose of halothane; experience is
the best guide there. At the end of the operation the residual effects of curare, Pavolon or gallamine can be reversed by an acetyl-cholinesterase inhibitor
such as neostigmine. However, neostigmine is only effective if some muscle
function is already present. Too large and too late doses of relaxants should
therefore be avoided. As neostigmine is a vagostimulant it must be combined
with atropine (Vagolytica).

Dosage: 0.03 mg neostigmine/kg body wt. +0.01 atropine/kg body wt. IV.

I.P.P.V. should be continued during the period of reversal until neuromuscular function has fully returned. An increase of CO_2 during this period
of reversal can lead to arrhythmia and sudden cardial arrest. Ventilate the

patient well, keep your finger on the pulse and remember that neostigmine takes 5 min to develop its peak effect.

Do not attempt to remove the tube too early when there is inadequate ventilation — keep on ventilating. If you are sure that respiration is fully established again, give if possible additional O_2 for some minutes. This will also help to avoid a laryngospasm during extubation. Suck out all mucus from the trachea and pharynx, but insert the suction catheter without sucking; *use suction only while withdrawing!* Ventilate 2-3 times again, deflate the cuff and remove, while sucking the tube gently in the expiratory period. Check if the patient is breathing well and that there is no airway obstruction. Observe him for 3-5 min and leave your patient only when you are absolutely sure that he is in full control of his respiration and that he responds to stimuli and reacts to being called.

A prolonged recovery period may be caused by:

a) Inadequate oxygenation during anaesthesia and the recovery period (respiratory acidosis). Treatment consists of hyperventilation but *no* Na HCO_3 (sodium bicarbonate).
b) Metabolic acidosis, e.g. after cardiac arrest or impaired maintenance of circulation. Treatment consists of 50-100 ml Na HCO_3 8.4% solution, IV +infusion, even blood.
c) Antibiotics

Streptomycin, neomycin, polymycin are antibiotics which may produce curare-like effects. They should not be given during or shortly before an operation. If they are given and a delay of reversal is observed, give 10 ml 10% calcium gluconate slowly IV. *The best treatment of prolonged apnea is adequate ventilation.*

Name: Age: BW:

	History	Clinicl. Examination	Remarks/Drugs
Resp. system			
C. V. S.			
HGL.	Urine	Remarks	
Date:	Premedication		
Time:			
Relax			
Inhalation			Intubation
			System
200			Time
180			
160			Complications
140			
120			
100			
80			
60			
40			
20			

Post op treatment

Chapter 8

Anaesthesia in Obstetrics

Certain factors dominate the technique of performing anaesthesia in obstetrics:

There are two human beings in one, but anaesthesia should only effect one; the presence of abdominal distention; and the presence or absence of foetal distress. Therefore in performing anaesthesia in obstetrics it is necessary to use anaesthetic drugs with little or no effect on the foetus.

8.1 Drugs

Narcotics which do not pass the placenta perial or have very little effect on the foetus and can therefore be used in obstetric anaesthesia include the following:

a) Thiopentone: up to 250 mg IV. Thiopentone crosses the placenta immediately, but the concentration of the barbiturate in the foetus falls as time elapses and the drug is metabolised by the mother. Therefore, the longer the time (4-5 min) from injection until the child is delivered, the less the effect.

b) Epontol: 0.5 g IV. Epontol is very quickly metabolised and has no notable effects.

c) Ketalar: 2 mg/kg body wt. or as a drip. Ketalar has very little effect on the foetus.

d) N_2O+O_2 (2:1). Gas and air has no effect on the foetus.

Muscle relaxants which may be used:

Scoline 1 mg/kg body wt. (very quickly metabolised, no effect). Curarine crosses the placenta in amounts sufficient to affect the foetus and should only be used for relaxation of the mother *after the baby is delivered.*

Flaxedil has exactly the same effects as curarine and the same conditions therefore apply.

8.2 Adequate O₂ Tension

Impaired O$_2$ tension and hypotension cause immediate danger to the foetus. Impaired O$_2$ tension is easily caused by abdominal distension and the danger of vomiting and also by respiratory depression from the anaesthetic drugs. Therefore administer O$_2$ substitute during induction. For anaesthesia under spontaneous respiration O$_2$ subsitute is essential.

Be prepared to manage vomiting (sucker, head down and quick intubation, see Fig. 8.1).

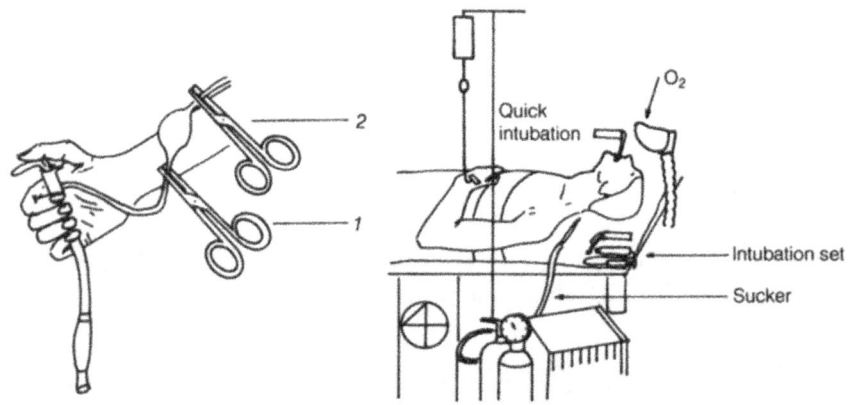

Fig. 8.1. Technique for quick intubation. First put forceps *1* after the pilot bulb, inflate the cuff and set forceps 2. As soon as you have intubated, open forceps *1*, so that the air from the pilot bulb will inflate the cuff

Hypotension and inadequate IV fluid in the mother, will all cause impaired blood supply to the placenta and therefore will endanger the baby. Efforts must be made to maintain adequate BP by sufficient infusion therapy.

Prepare everything necessary for proper anaesthesia. Do not forget atropine. Give good pre-anaesthetic oxygenation.

8.3 General Anaesthesia for Caesarean Section

Premedication:	0.5 mg atropine IM or IV
Induction:	500 mg Epontol IV or 200 mg thiopentone IV
Relaxation:	1 mg Scoline/kg body wt. IV
Intubation:	IPPR maintenance of amnesia, 6%-4% ether or O_2 +N_2O and halothane

If more relaxation is needed, give 20 mg Scoline IV until the child is born. After delivery maintain relaxation with curarine or any other muscle relaxant. If spontaneous respiration is wanted use no further relaxants and maintain anaesthesia with ether or O_2+N_2O and halothane. *During Caesarean section the mother loses much blood. Set up an IV drip before anaesthesia and give adequate fluid.*

Sometimes a brief anaesthesia is required to reduce pain and to increase relaxation. If only a very short anaesthesia is required 500 mg Epontol IV is the answer. If, however, longer anaesthesia is needed, e.g. for a forceps or breech delivery, the Ketalar drip, with or without a relaxant, is a very useful technique (see Chap. 10).

8.4 Care and Resuscitation of the Neonatal

The condition of the baby can be assessed by ascertaining the factors in Table 8.1. Note: Record the Apgar after 1 and 5 min. For example, on delivery points might be calculated as: respiration, regular=2; heartbeat, 120=2; muscle tonus, moderate=1; reflexes, fair=2; Apgar Sc.=8.

Table 8.1

Respiration	Heartrate	Mus. tonus	Colour	Reflexes	Notes
Regular	120	strong	normal	+	good=2
Gasping	100	moderate	slight blue	weak	fair=1
Apnea	80	flaccid	grey	—	bad=0

8-10 points: Clean the airway and keep warm.
6-8 points: Clean airway and assist breathing with ambubag.
1-5 points: Use the following system: A.B.C.D.

A. *Airway cleared by sucking*
First mouth, then nose. No endotracheal – sucking without IPPR afterwards.
B. *Breathing*
       1) Ambubag
Breathing
       2) Intubation   *Does the air reach the lung?*
C. *Circulation*
External heart massage
D. *Drugs*
0.1 mg Alupent/kg body wt. Correction of acidosis: with 2 mVal Na HCO_3/ kg body wt.

Note: Na HCO_3 without ventilation

Note also: If the mother has been given pethedine within 4 h of delivery, and if the baby is not doing well, it should be given *Nalorphan.*

Chapter 9
Paediatric Anaesthesia

In anaesthesia children should not be considered small adults.

The physical difference between children and adults is derived from six major points:

1) *High metabolic rate*
The metabolic O_2 requirements of the neonatal is 7 ml/kg body wt. compared to 3.5 ml/kg body wt. in adults. This means a child can go blue in half the time. Furthermore, the metabolic rate in a child goes up in high temperatures. Therefore a good O_2 supply of at least 50% during anaesthesia should be applied to avoid critical errors.

2) *Small volume of tidal air, large anatomical dead space, rapid respiratory rate*
The anatomical dead space in neonatals, in comparison to the alveolar ventilating air, is greater than in adults. This is easily understood by remembering that tidal air in the neonatal is only 19 ml. In order to meet its high oxygen requirements with its small tidal air, the respiratory rate is much more rapid.

3) *Rapid circulation*
Anaesthetic drugs are quickly absorbed, act quickly, but are also much more quickly metabolised. Changes in the depth of anaesthesia in either direction occur more rapidly.

4) *Large surface area*
The smaller an object, the greater its surface area in comparison with its interior. Therefore a child under anaesthesia cools more rapidly than an adult. *Fall of temperature can be fatal to a child in its first year of life.*

5) *Differences in the airway structure*
There is a narrow passage, a relatively large tongue, high angled laryngeal cords and a narrow sub-glottic region.

6) *Less vagal tone*
There is a great risk of cardiac inhibition and laryngospasm.

9.1 Equipment

The choice of equipment has to be guided by a minimum resistance to respiration (e.g. heavy valves), a minimum dead space and a high O_2 flow. Our normal technical equipment (E.M.O. or Boyle's machine) is not suitable for children under 15 kg, because of the big dead space up to the valves; remember 19 ml. Anaesthesia should be performed with the so-called T-piece (see Fig. 9.1), or with smaller technical equipment. It is important to realise that there must be a fresh gas flow and not a source of fresh air.

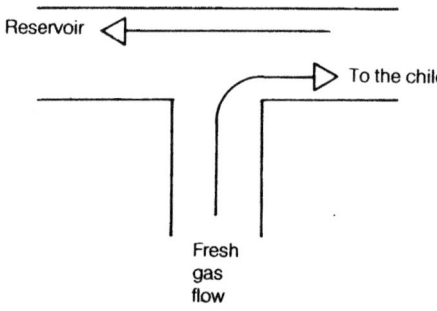

Reservoir

To the child

Fresh
gas
flow

Fig. 9.1

The Kuhn-Child Set is in principle the same as the T-piece and is a suitable unit (see Fig. 9.2).

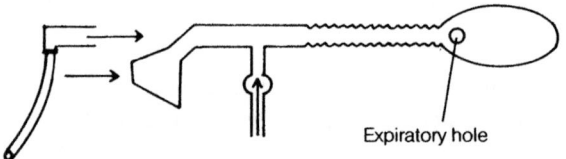

Expiratory hole

Fig. 9.2

There is no valve and a very small dead space, and it can be used for spontaneous respiration. Part of the gas is *blown* in from the fresh gas source and inhaled by the child, while expiratory air goes to the expiratory port or bag.

The fresh gas supply should be at least 200 ml/kg body wt/min. One half of it at least should be O_2. Too small a gas flow results in rebreathing if the volume of the expiratory part is greater than the patient's tidal volume. Controlled ventilation is required: the expiratory hole must be closed with the thumb, while the bag is squeezed rhythmically. The rate should be 30-40 times per min. The bag must never be allowed to over-distend and the thumb must only be over the expiratory hole for the inspiration.

9.2 Technique of Anaesthesia

A useful technique is the Ketalar-drip, intubation and ventilation as described in Chapter 10 only using the Ambu pediatric set. (Ambubag and paediatric valve).

9.2.1 Premedication and Induction

Premedication: see Chapter 4. For induction use 2 mg Ketalar/kg body wt. IM, with a machine with halothane gas or O_2 or 3 mg Penthotal/kg body wt. IV.

9.2.2 Intubation

Intubation can be carried out in deep anaesthesia or, ideally, under relaxation: 1 mg Scoline/kg body wt. The Mackintosh laryngoscope and endotracheal tube are recommended (see Chapter 5).

In the first few days of life or in very weak babies intubation may be performed without anaesthesia and relaxation. The baby should be firmly wrapped and held by an assistant. In infants the larynx is higher and the epiglottis longer, which might necessitate external pressure on the trachea to bring the cords into view. The Kuhn and the Oxford tubes are the most suitable ones. The Oxford tube has to be used with a stiletto to increase the curve of the tube. The stiletto is made from hard plastic and is placed 1/2 in. before the tubes level (see Fig. 9.3). Never insert a tube further than 1 in. below the cords. Use the largest of the tubes, which will *slip down easily*. Too small a tube will increase breathing resistance. All endotracheal tubes must be fixed firmly by strapping. Remember that in infants the tube can slip out easily.

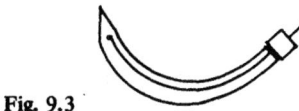

Fig. 9.3

9.2.3 Continuous Anaesthesia and Relaxation

The alternatives for general anaesthesia are: air-ether (Afya); O_2+N_2O+halothane or a Ketalar drip.

For relaxation, use a Scoline drip for short operations. Otherwise either 0.4 mg curarine/kg body wt. or 1 mg Flaxedil/kg body wt. For repeated doses give one-quarter of the initial dosage.

For the reversal of relaxants use 0.01 mg atropine/kg body wt. and 0.08 mg neostigmine/kg body wt.

9.2.4 Monitoring

In infants it is best to have a stethoscope strapped to the left chest (see Fig. 9.4). In this way you can listen to both the apex beat and the air entry into the left lung and thereby the ventilation and the heartbeat can easily be monitored. Also observe the colour of the blood and of the mucous membranes. Press the skin with your finger for an instant. The return of colour is an indication of good circulation.

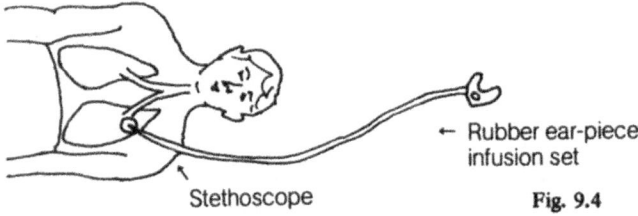

← Rubber ear-piece
infusion set

Stethoscope

Fig. 9.4

9.2.5 Recovery and Extubation

Before extubation be sure the normal neuromuscular function has returned. Give 100% O_2 or hyperventilate the child. Suck the pharynx, possibly with the help of a laryngoscope. Do not suck the trachea; but if you do, lay up I.P. P.R. again, and remove the tube. *Never leave the child alone even for one second!*

9.2.6 Prevention of Cooling

Always keep the child warm with cloth-covered hot-water bottles. Wrap as much as possible of the baby in a cotton sheet and bandage. Avoid wet sheets near the body of the baby. Undercooling of the baby will effect respiratory depression and metabolic acidosis and cause the failure of the reversal of muscle relaxants. The effect of undercooling may not be reversed; therefore strict prevention is the best safeguard. Undercooling may often cause fatality in neonatal anaesthesia. *Blood transfusion,* fluid and electrolytic balance during surgery. For maintenance of fluid and electrolysis use 0.18 NaCl in glucose, never use 0.9% NaCl in dextrose.

Pulse rate and volume are the best guide for adequate infusion and transfusion. In neonatals any blood loss over 30 ml should be replaced (preferably with a syringe). If the blood loss is more than 10% of the blood volume in older children, replace it.

Remember:

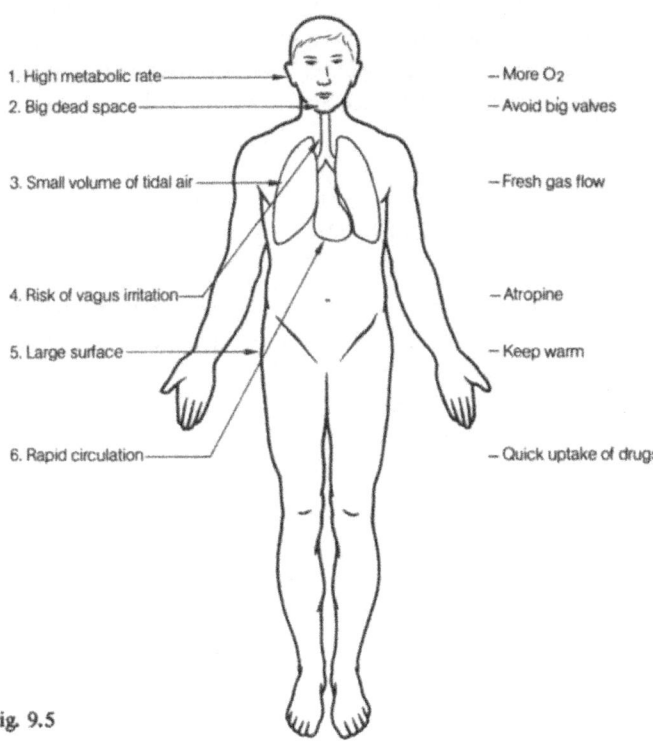

1. High metabolic rate — ... More O₂
2. Big dead space — — Avoid big valves
3. Small volume of tidal air — — Fresh gas flow
4. Risk of vagus irritation — — Atropine
5. Large surface — — Keep warm
6. Rapid circulation — — Quick uptake of drugs

Fig. 9.5

Chapter 10
Ketalar-Mono Anaesthesia

Ketalar-Mono Anaesthesia is a reliable and safe technique for various operations and surgical procedures. Very little technical equipment is required and this method is widely used, especially in developing countries. The technique provides either a short-acting anaesthesia with single or repeated doses or prolonged anaesthesia using Ketalar as a drip, with or without relaxation.

10.1 Short-Acting Anaesthesia

Premedication: 0.1-0.2 mg haloperidol/kg body wt. at least
            1 h before the operation, atropine 0.01 mg/kg i.m. 1/2 h
            before the operation
Induction: 2 mg Ketalar/kg body wt.
            1-2 min before operation.
Control: B P, pulse and respiration

If further anaesthesia is required give half of the initial dosage again IV. After surgery put the patient in quiet surroundings in the coma position and under observation until fully recovered.

This technique can be used for the opening and drainage of an abscess, the reduction of a fracture, painful dressings and D and C.

10.2 Anaesthesia for Longer than 20 Minutes

Ketalar-drip anaesthesia is more suitable for longer surgical procedures. It is necessary to emphasise that equipment for resuscitation and a blood pressure machine should be present. An Ambubag or other ventilator, endotracheal intubation equipment and a simple foot-sucker should be at hand.

Premedication: 0.1 mg haloperidol/kg body wt., atropin 0.01 mg/kg body wt.

A good and reliable peripheric needle for a drip should be set up. Ketalar is given as a solution: 500 ml dextrose containing 500 mg Ketalar, i.e. 1 ml dextrose to 1 mg Ketalar.

Induction: Start the drip off at a rate of 100-160 drops/min. (Roughly 2 drops/min/kg body wt.)

In the pre-surgical stage the patient develops a vacant stare, does not respond to pain but still has reflexes, e.g. eyelashes, corneal, pharyngeal.

Maintenance: once the surgical state has been reached, the drip rate is reduced to 60-80 drops/min (1 drop/min/kg body wt.). Respiration, pulse rate and B P are monitored throughout anaesthesia. 5-7 min before the end of surgery, the anaesthesia drip is stopped.

10.3 Indication and Technique

Ketalar-Mono is suitable in any case not requiring deep muscular relaxation or the deadening of reflexes, e.g. operations on extremities and reconstructive surgery.

The technique is simple and when applied with normal intelligence, relatively safe; necessary equipment is minimal. The major disadvantage is the poor muscular relaxation; for this, the technique can be modified by Ketalar drip relaxant and artificial respiration.

The equipment required:

1) Infusion set
2) Ambubag-Ambu "E" valve (and air)
3) Laryngoscope with suitable blades
4) Range of endotracheal tubes
5) Suction and catheters
6) Elephant-tubing
7) Drugs: Infusion (Ringer-Lactate)
            Ketalar
            Scoline
            Curarine or Flaxedil
            atropine
            neostigmine

Premedication: 0.1 mg haloperidol/kg body wt., 1 h before operation.

Induction: Administer Ketalar-drip up to 100 drops/min. As soon as the patient loses consciousness reduce the drip to 30-40 drops/min (1/2 mg Ketalar/min/kg body wt.). To intubate patient give 1 mg Scoline/kg body wt. Following intubation, respiration is maintained with the ambubag and atmospheric air. As soon as neuromuscular function returns a non-depolarising relaxant is given, e.g. 0.2 mg d-tubocurarine/kg body wt. or gallamine triethiodide=Flaxedil 1-2 mg/kg body wt. Artificial respiration is maintained by squeezing the bag. A comfortable squeeze of the bag yields 500 ml and the aim is a minute volume of=1 litre per 10 kg body wt./min.

Reversal: 10-15 min before the end of the operation the Ketalar-drip is stopped, but ventilation is continued.

Give 0.01 mg atropine/kg body wt. and then 0.02 mg neostigmine/kg body wt. IV.

Continue ventilation until the return of adequate neuromuscular function. Extubation is then performed in the usual way. For those requiring IV fluid or blood during the operation, have a separate drip for this purpose. (For children under 14 kg use the paediatric Ambubag for ventilation.)

The technique described above demonstrates the essential requirements of good anaesthesia; good analgesia, hypnosis and muscular relaxation without undesirable side-effects.

Ketalar produces a profound state of analgesia and light amnesia with a quick recovery period. A muscle relaxant provides adequate relaxation while atmospheric air (usually) provides enough oxygen.

The choice of haloperidol for premedication is of some importance. Haloperidol balances or cancels most of the important side-effects of Ketalar. The hypertension described with the use of Ketalar in some reports does not occur very frequently, due to the alpha-receptor-blocking effect of haloperidol. Swings of B P and pulse rate are much reduced, compared to the sole use of Ketalar, and in our opinion mild degrees of hypertension do not contraindicate the use of Ketalar-drip, when haloperidol is used too (see Fig. 10.1). The often-reported hallucinations or bad dreams are much lessened by the use of this premedication. The increase of saliva production can pose a problem and might make frequent sucking necessary. Most significant is the wide margin of safety. Sources of error, technical or human, are reduced to a minimum (see Fig. 10.2 a,b).

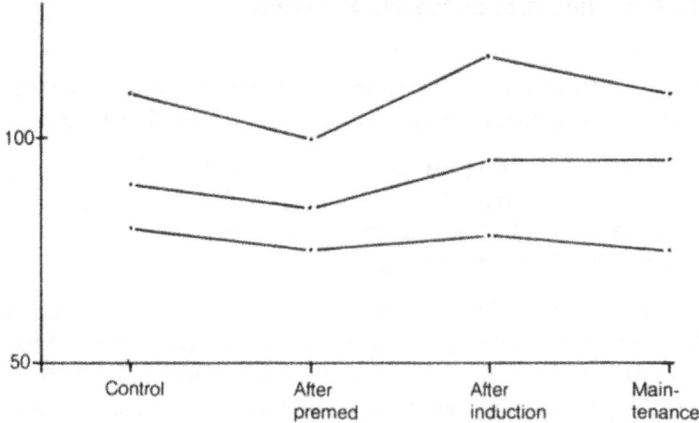

100 —

50 —

Control | After premed | After induction | Maintenance

Fig. 10.1

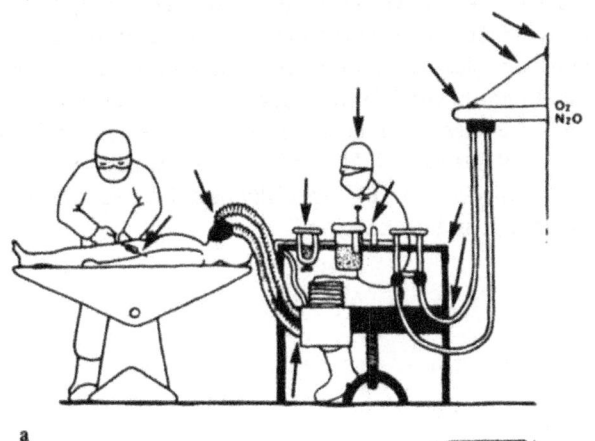

a

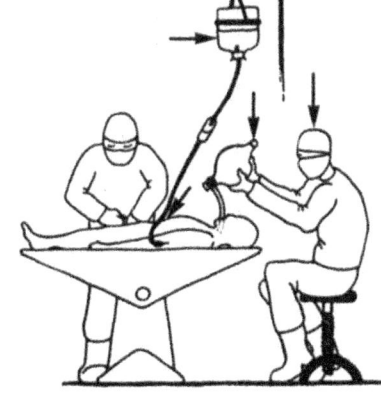

Fig. 10.2. a Possible human and technical sources of error with the usual complex methods of anaesthesia; b Possible human and technical sources of error with anaesthetic ketamine drip and relaxant. Note: The addition of a length of elephant tubing between Ambubag and Ambu "E" valve gives the anaesthetist very great freedom of movement and can be recommended

b

10.4 Scoline-drip as Muscle Relaxant

For short surgical procedures, where optimal relaxation is needed air-ether-E.M.O. anaesthesia, using the Scoline-drip as a muscle relaxant is reliable.

Technique: 0.01 mg atropine/kg body wt. IM +haloperidol or pethedine
              as hypnotic
Induction: 0.3-0.5 mg thiopentone/kg body wt.
Relaxation: ` 1 mg Scoline/kg body wt.

Intubation and I.P.P.R.: inhalation-anaesthesia e.g. ether or halothane. After the first *reliable sign of neuromuscular activity,* start off the Scoline-drip: 500 mg Scoline in 500 ml dextrose 5% (1ml/1mg), 10-30 drops/min according to the lung condition and muscular relaxation. Continue I.P.P.R. using the inhalation anaesthetic agent only as a hypnotic (ether 3%-4%, halothane 0.5%-1%). At the end of the operation stop the Scoline-drip and anaesthesia, continuing ventilation until full respiration and reflex activity are returned. Clean the airway and extube in the usual manner. This technique should not be used for long operations or exceed the dosage of 500 mg Scoline. The advantage lies in quick recovery of the patient from anaesthesia and relaxation. While using E.M.O. ether-air-anaesthesia the Scoline-drip is easy, cheap and relatively safe. It is especially useful for tonsillectomies and operations in the mouth and neck region.

Chapter 11
Anaesthesia for Ophthalmic Surgery

The choice of anaesthesia for ophthalmic surgery is influenced by two major factors:

1. Optimal relaxation of the eye, including post-operative condition, is absolutely necessary.
1.1. It is nearly impossible to perform a neat and tiny operation on a moving subject.

Coughing, Vomiting and Pressing can Cause Bleeding and Prolapse of the Vitredus Leading to Irreparable Damage

2. Reduction of the intra-ocular pressure is requested.
2.1. A lowered intra-ocular pressure and tension *is* required for intra-ocular operation (vitreous prolapse), a normal tension for extra capsular lens extraction.

Therefore it is Important that the Intra-ocular Pressure (i.o.p.) should not be unduly raised by anaesthesia.

The intra-ocular pressure is raised by:

1) Hypoxaemia
2) Hypoventilation
3) Coughing
4) Top light anaesthesia
5) Excitation stage during and after ophthalmic anaesthesia
6) Epontol
7) Ketalar
8) Scoline (Suxamethonium)

The intra-ocular pressure is lowered by:

1) Hyperventilation
2) Hyperoxaemia
3) Ether, Halothane, Penthrane, Trichloroethylene
4) Neuroleptica

5) Hypnotica, e.g. Barbiturates
6) Non-depolarising relaxants
7) Dehydration
8) Deep anaesthesia

Premedication

The Success of Anaesthesia in Ophthalmic Surgery Depends to a Considerable Extent on the Proper Administration of Premedication

The existence of the oculocardiac reflex is well known and presents a serious complication for ophthalmic anaesthesia. Bradycardia as well as tachycardia causes mechanical irritation on the bulbus and annexes. Atropine and adequate anaesthesia has a protective effect on the oculocardiac reflex.

Atropine, however, raises the i.o.p. only in the presence of glaucoma with a narrow angle between the cornea and iris, a genetically determined state.

Dosage: 0.01 mg/kg atropine intramuscularly (i.m.) 30 min before operation.

The pre- and post-operative sedation of the patient is necessary in ophthalmic surgery.

Premedication should also contribute to the post-operative tranquillity of the patient. Complications in ophthalmic surgery are often a result of poor pre-operative sedation.

The existence of fear before the operation as well as the psychological stress of an operation under local anaesthesia requires that the patient be adequately sedated. Heavy sedation, however, should be avoided, especially in older people. The so-called neuroleptica have proved to be suitable premedicative agents, mainly because of the good sedative effect, strong anti-emetic effect and long duration plus low toxicity.

2.2. Premedication with neuroleptica produces a calm drowsiness and lessening of anxiety. It should be noted that this sleep is in no way comparable to that induced by the usual hypnotics. The patient can still be awakened and after he has been informed of what is going on, he is allowed to return to sleep.

In general we noticed a slight falling of the arterial tension which could be the result of the alpha-receptor-blocking effect of the drug as well as a slowing down of the pulse rate.

2.3. With regard to respiratory system, the amplitude as well as the frequency are not affected by haloperidol administered in normal therapeutic dosages.

Besides, haloperidol or droperidol have an anti-emetic effect – to avoid post-operative vomiting after anaesthesia. Haloperidol is mostly available. It can be used even in combination with Valium (our standard technique).

Haloperidol   0.1 mg/kg per os or i.m. 1 1/2 or 1 h before op.
Valium   0.2 mg/kg

Haloperidol requires 1-1 1/2 h to become fully active; the duration is 12 h.
Therefore the premedication can be given to all respective patients at the same time in the morning.

Anaesthetic Techniques

3. *Local Anaesthesia*

Most of the ophthalmic operations can and should be performed under local anaesthesia. This should thus be aimed at and is possible with good premedication. The only real contraindications for local anaesthesia are very long-lasting operations and ophthalmic surgery in children.
Advantages of local anaesthesia:

1. Safer
2. Less interference with the normal physiology
3. Less post-operative complications

Disadvantages

1. Lack of control of the patient (premedication)
2. Operations lasting a long time are difficult to perform
3. Unsuitable for children

Conduction Anaesthesia for Intra-ocular Surgery

Eyelid Paresis can be achieved by anaesthetising the m. orbicularis oculi according to the method of van Lint.
This is necessary prior to all intra-ocular surgery, in order to prevent blepharospasm which can endanger the success of the operation. The needle is inserted at right angles to the skin until the lower lateral angle of the inferior orbital margin is reached. Here, with the tip of the needle against the edge of the bone, 1 ml of a 2% solultion of lignocaine or prilocaine with vasoconstrictor is injected.
The needle is then redirected and 2 ml of the same solution are injected along the lateral margin of the orbit.

Still from the same point of insertion another 2 ml of the solution are injected along the inferior orbital margin.

Retrobulbar Anaesthesia

Anatomy

The ciliary ganglion, measuring 2-3 mm in length, lies deep in the orbit just lateral to the optic nerve and medial to the lateral rectus muscle. Immediately behind the ganglion, the ophthalmic artery winds around the lateral side of the optic nerve and crossing above it passes forwards in a medial direction.

Technique

The needle used should be exactly 3.5 cm long or alternatively should bear a marker at this distance from its point, so as to reach the ciliary ganglion but at the same time avoiding the risk of puncturing the blood vessels in the apex of the orbit.

The injection is performed through the lower eyelid, at the lower lateral angle of the orbit. During the insertion of the needle the patient should look upwards and medially, which produces a contraction of the inferior oblique muscle and allows the needle to pass under it more easily.

The anterior part of the eye is moved away from the needle in order to gain better access to the ciliary ganglion.

The lower lateral angle of the orbit is palpated. The needle is inserted through the skin, where 0.5 ml of plain 2% solution of lignocaine or prilocaine is injected. The needle is directed towards the apex of the orbit, i.e. backwards, inwards and upwards.

Slowly and while injecting simultaneously 0.5-1.0 ml of solution (in order to replace any blood vessel along the path of the needle) the needle is inserted in its entire length or alternatively up to the marker, i.e. exactly 3.5 cm. Careful aspiration is essential to exclude the possibility of an intravenous injection.

Then 1.5-2 ml of a plain 2% solution of lignocaine or prilocaine are administered, taking 5-10 s over the injection.

If complete akinesia is desired, the volume injected may be increased to 4 ml. After removal of the needle, 5 ml should be allowed to slapse before surgery is commenced.

Normal Response

The pupil dilates, and the intra-ocular pressure is reduced. Partial or total paralysis of the extrinsic muscles of the eye is achieved.

Retrobulbar anaesthesia always produces slight exophthalmus, directly proportioned to the volume injected. The recommended volume of 1.5-2 ml is adequate for the majority of intra-ocular procedures, but larger doses, (at least 4 ml) are recommended for enucleation, or for the photo- or electrocoagulation of the retina.

Complications

Retrobulbar haematoma. This rarely occurs unless the needle is inserted for more than 3.5 cm. If a haematoma should form, it always does so within 5 min of the injection. In such a case the operation is deferred until the exophthalmus has regressed. If exophthalmus is marked a pressure dressing is applied.

Paralysis of the Superior Rectus Muscle

Frequently the patient will still be able to move the eyeball upwards to a certain extent. Since this may be a disadvantage in intra-ocular surgery, retrobulbar anaesthesia may have to be augmented by anaesthesia of the superior rectus muscle.

The patient is asked to look downwards, and the upper eyelid is retracted, a 2 cm long needle is inserted into Tenon's capsule (fascia bulbi) at the lateral edge of the superior rectus muscle and 1 ml lignocaine or prilocaine 1.0% with vasoconstrictor is injected into the belly of the muscle, posterior to the equator of the eyeball.

4. General Anaesthesia

Advantages

1. Less of an ordeal for the patient (especially if no premedication)
2. The patient is quiet, *especially children*
3. More suitable for long operations
4. Suitable conditions for the surgeon (quiet, quick)

General Aspects

Except for really short procedures, where a short mask anaesthesia is performed in general anaesthesia, the patient should be intubated to ensure proper maintenance and ventilation of the airway.

For longer operations relaxation and J.P.P.V. is recommended. Any long operation is unsuitable for local anaesthesia and should be done under general anaesthesia.

Remember Hypoxia – Hypoventilation cause an increase in i.o.p.

A required fall of i.o.p. can be achieved by hyperventilation

Drugs and Technique Use for Central Anaesthesia

1. Barbiturates, useful for induction only, reduce i.o.p., cause hyperventilation
2. Ketalar – see Mono-Anaesthesia
3. Ether: good drug for anaesthesia but causes respiratory tract irritation and vomiting. – Premedication!
4. *Relaxants:* Tubocurarine and gallamine lower the i.o.p.; may cause bradycardia.

Suxamethonium

Increases the i.o.p., but the rise is probably confined to the period of apnoea (proper technique). There is no reason for banning this useful aid for intubation and relaxation. It should, however, never be used as the first drug during the operation, when the eye is already open, for fear of precipitating vitreous prolapse.

The Halfopen E.M.O. Ether-Air-Anaesthetic-Technique

is safe, simple and cheap. Besides, the E.M.O. anaesthetic machine is often available in developing countries.

Some Suitable General Anaesthetic Techniques

Premedication

Haloperidol	0.1 mg/kg per os	
Valium	0.1 mg/kg " " at least 1 h before op.	
atropine	0.01 mg/kg i.m. 1/2 h before op.	

Induction

    Intravenous   Thiopental 3-5 mg/kg i.v.
                         Suxamethonium 1 mg/kg i.v.

Endotracheal Intubation – Ventilation

The topical analgesia of the larynx and trachea with a 4% solution of lignocaine is in most cases helpful. It can be applied easily, e.g. with a Macintosh spray or astra-lignocaine spray before intubation. This will make it easier for the amount of anaesthetic drugs to be reduced (the endotracheal tube is more irritating than the pain from the operation) as well as coughless extubation.

Spontaneous respiration is advised only for operations under 30 min. Set ether concentration on around 10%. Ventilate the patient until spontaneous respiration returns. Usually by the time the spontaneous respiration returns, the patient will breathe quietly and is ready for surgery. The ether concentration can then be reduced to maintenance level of 6%-8%.

The patient should be ventilated adequately, but hyperventilation will prolonge the return of spontaneous respiration.

Hypoventilation, however, will lead to more serious complications.

If relaxation is to be maintained by the use of a muscle relaxant (for long-lasting operations) ether or whatever drug is used as an inhalating anaesthetic agent is only used to achieve hypnosis.

Muscle relaxation is produced by the adding of a muscle relaxing drug: e.g. Flaxedil (gallamine) 2 mg/kg or using the Scoline-drip.

After induction and intubation, ether concentration is set on 4% volume-, ventilation – and as soon as the neuromuscular function returns (moving of lips), relaxation is maintained by giving preferably a long-acting muscle relaxant as mentioned above.

After the start of the operation and settling down of the patient, e.g. easy ventilation, the ether concentration can be reduced to 3%-4% to maintain amnesia. As soon as relaxation becomes inadequate and the operation is not to be finished soon, give 1/2 of the initial dosage of muscle relaxant again.

Recovery Period

It is important that the extubation as well as the recovery period is as smooth as possible. This means that the anaesthesia should not be stopped too early and that the extubation has to be performed still "in anaesthesia" to avoid coughing.

If reversal of the muscle relaxant is necessary give

atropine 0.01 mg/kg +neostigmine 0.03 mg/kg i.v. and

continue to ventilate until spontaneous respiration returns. If possible, suck the mouth only and extubate very carefully. *Make sure the patient breathes well!*

Monitoring

I. Ventilation

Fresh gas	—	Adequate ventilation	—	Chest movement
Anaesthetic concentration				Colour of blood
Correct gas mixture	*Volume*	*Frequency*		Colour of nails
	10 ml/kg	12-18 Adults		and skin
	per frequency	25-30 Children		

II. Circulation

Pulse — if normal — keep it

Bradycardia
↓
Vagus —
CO_2
O_2

Tachycardia
↓
atropine —
CO_2
O_2
Volume deficit

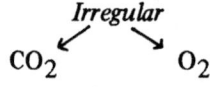

Irregular
CO_2 ← → O_2
Adrenaline + Halothane

III. Blood Pressure — if adequate — keep it

Hypertension
↓
Too light anaesthesia

Hypotension
↓
Too deep anaesthesia
Fall of O_2

Many studies do not recommend Scoline for ophthalmic surgery; but recent studies show that the increase in i.o.p. is more affected by the level of ventilation. We have used the Scoline-drip for relaxation and steadied the i.o.p., which did not show any significant changes, if proper premedication and ventilation is administered. The advantages are quick and smooth recovery from anaesthesia and relaxation occur.

Technique

Premedication — atropine — Haloperidol

Induction — relaxation — intubation — in the usual way.

After the first reliable sign of neuromuscular activity, start of the Scoline-drip — 500 mg Scoline in 500 ml of NaCl 0.9%, e.g. 1 ml = 1 mg. Speed of the drip according to the lung compliance and relaxation continuation and I.P.P.V. using the intubation anaesthetic agent only as a hypnotic, e.g. ether 3%-4% (quick recovery) and monitoring of the patient.

At the end of the operation, stop Scoline-drip, continue ventilation — assisted ventilation — until full respiration returns — cleaning of airway — extubation, as mentioned above, still under anaesthesia. This technique should not be used, however, for longer operations or exceed the dosage of 500 mg Scoline.

Ketalar-Mono-Anaesthesia has been used as a single anaesthetic agent, but advantages as well as disadvantages should be carefully considered:

Advantages
1. Relatively simple and easy
2. Relatively safe
3. A good anaesthetic technique, especially in children

Disadvantages
1. Expensive
2. Increase in i.o.p.
3. Relaxation not good, if Ketalar mono anaesthesia is used.

Relaxation of the Eye can be Improved by Using Local Anaesthesia

The so called dissociative anaesthesia presents a different form of anaesthesia. The reflex of swallowing as well as the tonus of the jaw and tongue is present, so that a free airway is usually being maintained. The respiration does not show major changes.

The cardiovascular system shows an increase in B P (10%-15%) and pulse rate. Also there is an increase in intra-ocular pressure (i.o.p.).

Frequent psycho-motoric changes often occur as an uncomfortable side-effect especially during the recovery period. This can, however, be diminished by the use of premedication (haloperidol, valium).

The frequent bulbus movements are very disturbing for the surgeon; they can, however, be checked by setting of a retrobulbar block.

Technique:

Do not forget premedication: Haloperidol, Valium per os. (atropine i.m.)

Induction by Ketalar-drip

500 mg Ketalar in 500 ml 0.18% NaCl via a reliable i.v. needle at a rate of 100-160 drops per min. until surgical stage is reached:

The patient develops a vacant stare – he does not respond to pain – but still has reflexes, e.g. eyelashes.

Set of the local anaesthetic retrobulbar block with lignocaine/adrenaline 1:10 000 (reduces also the bleeding tendency).

The drip rate then can be reduced to 60-80 drops per min= 1 drop min kg/B W. Respiration, pulse rate and B P are monitored throughout anaesthesia. 5-7 min before the end of the operation the anaesthesia drip is stopped. This technique is very useful, especially for children up to 7 years, since the E.M.O. Ether – Air – Technique cannot be used under 15 kg B W. If good relaxation is required or the operation is to last longer, this method should be used with relaxant and artificial ventilation, using a paediatric Ambu valve and bag for children and a normal bag for adults.

Technique
Premedication

atropine 0.01 mg/kg i.m. 1/2 h before op.
Haloperidol + Valium per os 1 " "   "

Set the i.v. Ketalar-drip and start at a quick speed until patient loses consciousness. Then the drip is reduced to 1/2 mg/kg/min for relaxation 1 mg/kg Scoline.

Intubation, artificial ventilation with the paediatric Ambubag and valve. As soon as neuromuscular function returns, a non-depolarising mucle relaxant is given, e.g. Flaxedil 1 mg/kg or d– tubocurarine 0.2 mg/kg. Artificial ventilation with Ambubag and air.

The Ketalar-drip is kept running to maintain amnesia.

Monitoring of the patient pref. extrath. stethoscope.

Reversal

Ten min before the end of the operation, the Ketalar-drip is stopped, but ventilation is kept up.

If reversal muscle relaxation is required:

atropine 0.01 mg/kg
Neostigmine 0.03 mg/kg

Ventilate until full return of adequate spontaneous ventilation occurs. Suction and extubation.

Chapter 12

Anaesthesia and Associated Medical Problems

12.1 Anaemia

Remember that with a haemoglobin of 3 g% a cardiac output of 6 litres leaves no safety margin at all. Patients with chronic anaemia have to be transfused slowly to avoid heart failure by anoxia weakened myocardium. Where there is no time to correct a low haemoglobin, give maximum oxygen during anaesthesia, replace blood steadily and aim at controlled ventilation – I.P.P.V. The anaemic patient withstands hypotension very badly, so avoid: Pentothal, spinal-anaesthesia; preferably use Ketalar.

12.2 Sickle Cell Anaemia

Sickling may be produced by low oxygen tensions or by acidosis. If general anaesthesia is given, maintain the oxygenation of the blood and the cardiac output. The technique is similar to that in anaemic patients; in addition, the patient may be rendered alkalotic by the administration of 8.4% solution of 2-3 mEq $NaHCO_3$/kg body wt. IV 2 h before anaesthesia.

12.3 Heart Disease

Patients with compensated heart diseases (their daily activity is not unduly limited) who have a mild dyspnea on exertion should not present great problems provided that hypoxia and hypotension are avoided. These patients are best managed with light anaesthesia (ether-air-Afya), a relaxant and controlled respiration. Additional oxygen should be given. Avoid anaesthetic drugs which have a negative impact on the myocardium.

Patients in heart failure require pre-anaesthetic treatment:
e.g. bed rest and digoxin diuretics.

In an emergency, where surgery is prior to the medical problem, similar to compensated heart diseases provide good oxygenation (I.P.P.V.). During surgery these patients should be given small quantities of salt solutions; dextrose is better. Blood loss should be replaced with whole blood as these patients already suffer from a salt and water overload.

12.4 Hypertension

Patients whose hypertension has been controlled with drugs present less problems than those with uncontrolled hypertension. Therefore, if a patient requires treatment for hypertension this is best started at once and the BP stabilised before anaesthesia and surgery. The patient should take his medicine as usual. Induction of anaesthesia may produce severe *hypo*tension, which should be avoided as this can cause myocardial ischaemia. Thiopentone, given slowly, followed by ether air and controlled ventilation is probably the technique of choice.

12.5 Chest Disease

Where acute infection is present give general anaesthesia only in emergencies; local anaesthesia is preferable. If general anaesthesia is essential, use a light anaesthetic, muscle relaxation and frequent suction of the trachea. Aminophylline may be given, but if possible avoid atropine. Ketalar-drip mono-anaesthesia can be an alternative to avoid the risk of contamination of the anaesthetic equipment. Provide good post-operative analgesia: small doses often, rather than large doses eight hourly.

12.6 Chronic Chest Disease

Pre-operative treatment with bronchodilators, physiotherapy and antibiotics is indicated.

For general anaesthesia give a light anaesthesia and a relaxant. Curare should be avoided as it may cause a bronchospasm as a result of histamine release. If a bronchospasm occurs, give up to 500 mg aminophylline IV slowly and possibly 100-500 mg hydrocortisone IV.

12.7 Liver Disease

Jaundiced patients may have a low prothrombin level. Give vitamin K IM for some days pre-operatively. Nearly all anaesthetic agent depress the liver function; therefore dosages should be reduced. Light anaesthesia and good oxygenation are recommended. Patients with jaundice are often sensitive to Suxamethonium and may be resistant to curare. However, the use of muscle relaxants allows a light level of anaesthesia and is recommended. Ketalar, a small dosage of thiopentone and ether air are probably the drugs of choice..

12.8 Renal Disease

Remember that "most of the IV anaesthetic drugs are excreted by the kidneys, some even unchanged". Give preferably local anaesthesia or Ketalar and avoid thiopentone and Flaxedil.

12.9 Diabetes

If possible, local anaesthesia should be given. Diabetics controlled by tablets or diet present few problems under general anaesthesia if no oral food has been consumed. Avoid glucose infusions and omit the tablets on the day of operation. Where the patient is on insulin the blood sugar will rise during the operation but not excessively. Omit food, glucose and insulin until after surgery and then the patient can be *newly assessed.* With unstable diabetes the blood sugar has to be controlled and treated. If glucose is necessary, calculate that one unit of plain insulin neutralises 2g glucose. Add 20 units insulin to 500 ml dextrose. Ether and Ketalar cause a rise in blood sugar but the effect is minimal if light ether or Ketalar anaesthesia and a relaxant are given.

Chapter 13

Local Anaesthesia

The principal aim of anaesthesiology is to abolish pain and this can be achieved either by inducing unconsciousness with general anaesthesia (causing *analgesia*, *hypnosis* and *muscle relaxation*) or by local anaesthesia, preventing painful impulses from reaching the cortex of the brain by blocking the sensory nerve impulses from a localised area, causing *analgesia* and *muscle relaxation.*

13.1 Pharmacology

All the chemical agents which have come into use for blocking the nerve impulses have the same mode of action. In low concentrations they delay, and when present in higher concentrations completely prevent, the migration of ions across the nerve membranes, which is the normal transmission of nerve impulses (see Fig. 13.1). This blocking effect lasts as long as the concentration is high enough. As soon as the concentration goes down the nerve regains its normal function.

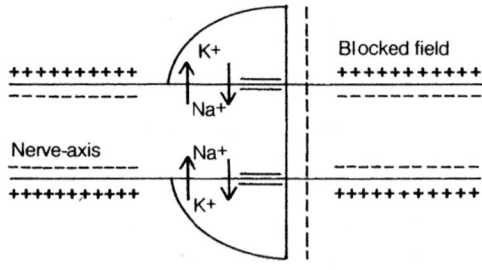

Fig. 13.1

The effect of local anaesthesia is largely dependent on the rate of perfusion and speed of absorption of the tissue. Reabsorption from the spinal cord is slow and consequently the duration of action is prolonged, while in the region of the jaw, for example, the action is so rapid that a vasoconstrictor has to be added to most local anaesthetics, if an adequate duration of action is to be obtained. Thin fibres are easier to block than coarse ones: a local anaesthetic with considerable power of penetration is required to block coarse nerve trunks. The stages of local anaesthesia are: loss of sensibility to pain, temperature (ether test), touch, and lastly, loss of motor function.

13.1.1 Addition of Vasoconstriction

The addition of a vasoconstrictor produces a localised vasoconstriction, delays reabsorption, prolongs the duration of action and reduces the risk of toxic side-effects. A vasoconstrictor, e.g. adrenaline, is added in a concentration of 1:200 000. In dental surgery only, concentrations of 1:80 000 are used.

Contraindications for the addition of a vasoconstrictor:

1) Tachycardiac patients
2) Technically on all peripheric areas: for instance, vasoconstriction in fingers would lead to ischaemia and necrosis. *(Never use a local anaesthetic with adrenaline in peripheric areas.)*

13.1.2 Toxicity

Local anaesthetic agents exert toxic effects if *they are absorbed into the general circulation* in sufficient concentrations. Toxic doses affect the C.N.S. by stimulation of the cerebral cortex, which results in tremors and convulsions. This may be explained by the fact that under normal conditions the inhibitory neurons in the cortex are most sensitive to the action of local anaesthetics. Consequently, blocking the inhibitory neurons would account for cortical excitation.

However, high concentrations inhibit the central neurons and depress the medulla, resulting in depression of the respiratory and cardio-vascular centres. Local anaesthetics also have a direct depression on the myocardium. However, cardiac arrhythmias can be treated with IV local anaesthetic. Different drugs vary widely in their toxicity and some people are consequently more sensitive to one compound than to another. The rate of injection, the quantity of drugs injected, the site of injection, the concentration of the local anaesthetic solution along with the age and the emotional and physical condition of the patient are factors which determine the development of toxic symptoms. It is a cardinal rule that the dosage of local anaesthetic should be kept as low as possible.

Maximum dosages:	
2% plain	10 ml
2% with adrenaline	25 ml
1% plain	20 ml
1% with adrenaline	50 ml
0.5% plain	40 ml
0.5% with adrenaline	100 ml

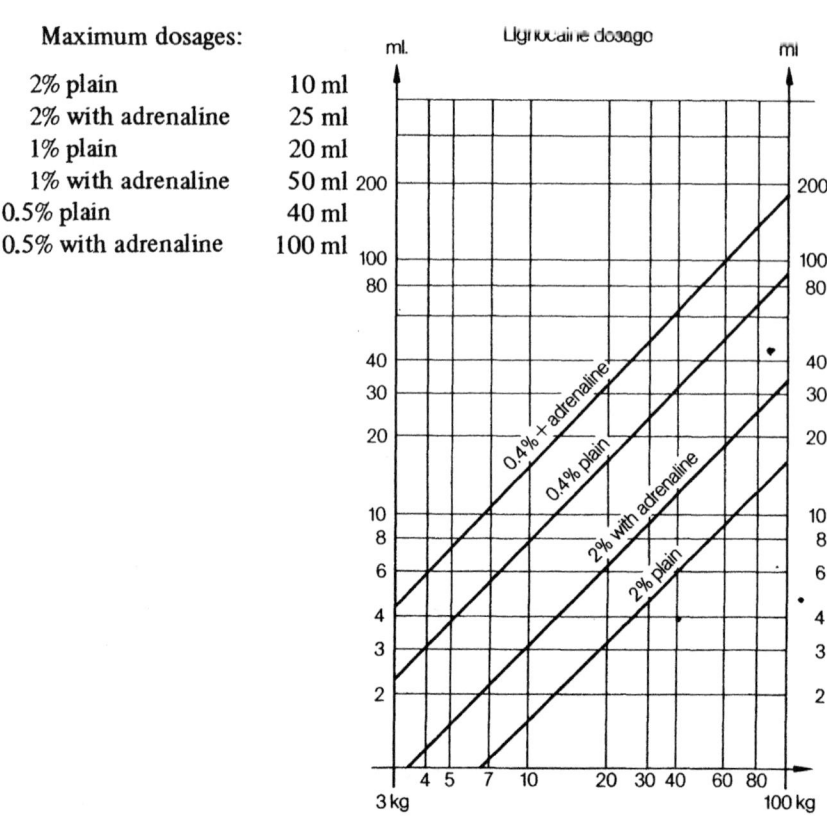

The interval between injections and development of action is 1-3 min. The duration of action is 1-3 h.

13.1.3 Metabolisation

Local anaesthetics are rapidly hydrolised in the plasma and in the liver to para-amino-benzoic acids and other chemical compounds and appear in the urine within 24 h.

13.2 Indications of Local Anaesthesia

1) Minor operations and small areas, operated with minimal interference of physiological mechanisms.

2) When it is desired to retain the co-operation of the patient during surgery or for patients who do not like to lose consciousness
3) Surgery where general anaesthesia would be too risky for the patient.
4) When an anaesthetist competent for general anaesthesia or devices for general anaesthesia are not available.

13.3 Complications

Either general or local complications may arise (see Table 13.1). There is also the possibility of allergic reaction to local anaesthetics with symptoms of shock.

Table 13.1

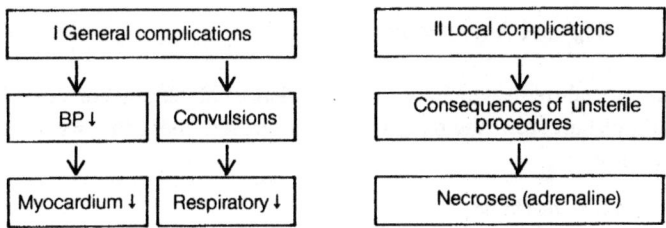

The appropriate actions to be taken, include the following:

Scheme of Treatment:
1) Treat *respiratory depression* with oxygen and artificial respiration via a mask or intubation
2) *Circulatory failure:* oxygen and the head-down position are recommended together with an infusion of a plasma-expander and appropriate drugs. Should cardiac arrest be suspected, commence external heart massage immediately.
3) *Convulsions:*

Give oxygen and a small dosage of barbiturate (1-2 mg/kg body wt. IV). If convulsions are severe succinyl-chlorine can be used to stop convulsions if the patient has lost consciousness and *is intubated.*

13.4 Types of Local Anaesthesia

13.4.1 Topical or Surface Anaesthesia

This is produced by an application of the drug directly on the surface of the skin or mucous membranes in order to produce loss of sensation by paralysing the affected nerve endings.

13.4.2 Infiltration Anaesthesia

Injectional drugs to block the nerve at the site of the proposed operation produce infiltration anaesthesia.

13.4.3 Regional Anaesthesia

The procedure in which a drug is applied to block a nerve along its source at a site distant from the region of the proposed operation. Regional anaesthesia includes:

a) *Spinal anaesthesia:*
   Introduced into the subarachnoid space in order to block the arterial and posterial routes and sympathetic fibres of nerves as they pass from the spinal cord through the space.
b) *Epidural anaesthesia:*
   Introduced into the epidural space.
c) *Nerve block:*
   Introduced to block a nerve at some points along the source before it divides into terminal branches (see Fig. 13.2).

13.5 Technique

Local anaesthesia should be performed with the same sterilisation precautions on the patient and the same technical equipment as those taken during surgical operations. Sterile syringes are required with two needles, one for the aspiration of the local anaesthesia and one for infiltration. The site of administration must be prepared and disinfected. For open wounds it is advisable to disinfect around the wound first, give local anaesthesia and after the analgetic

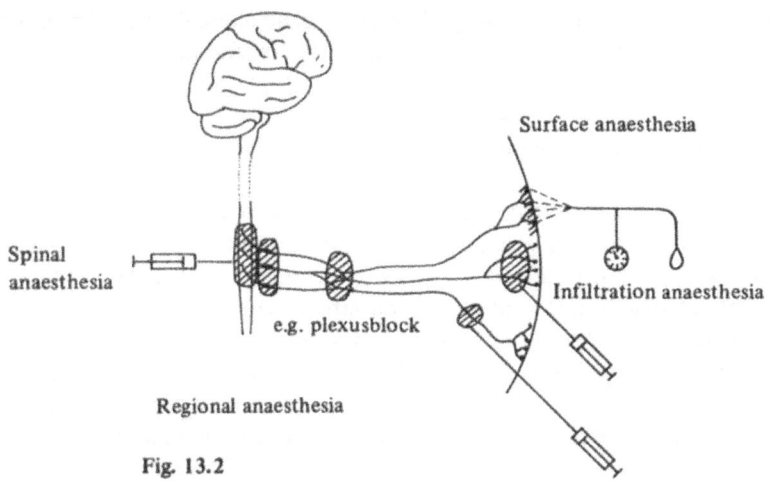

Surface anaesthesia

Spinal
anaesthesia

e.g. plexusblock

Infiltration anaesthesia

Regional anaesthesia

Fig. 13.2

effect is achieved, disinfect the whole area. It is a good routine in any local
anaesthesia to lay an indwelling IV needle on a peripheral vein in case of any
complications. Before infiltrations of higher amounts of local anaesthesia with
a big needle set a wheel first with a fine needle. Always remember, aspiration
in two directions is essential to avoid IV injection.

Many clinics consider the injection of local anaesthesia into infected tissue
to be contraindicated because of the danger of spreading bacteria in the sur-
rounding area. In tissue supplied by end arteries (toes, fingers, etc.), local anaesthesia solutions should be without vasoconstrictors.

13.5.1 Surface Anaesthesia

The anaesthetic is applied directly: to the skin; or to the mucous membranes
of the cornea or of the ear, nose and throat, or as a gel for the urethra. Where
the cornea is concerned, apply one drop for each installation; repeat after
1 min. This application of the anaesthetic agent may be used as a test of its
effect. For anaesthesia of the mucous membranes of the ear, nose or throat,
a concentration of 4% is used. Apply with a swab, syringe or with a local anaesthetic spray (Macintosh spray or similar).

In circumcision, put a ring of 1% lignocaine plain on the prepuce skin,
around where the outer skin cut is proposed (probably at the level of the corona at the base of the glands). Pull the foreskin back. Put another ring of 1%
plain round the inner prepuce skin, 4 mm behind the corona. Pull the foreskin
forward again. Wait for 5 min, then circumcise. If the prepuce cannot retract,

111

make a "dorsal slit", after running a line of 1% plain along the dorsal prepuce, back to the level of your first ring. Then make the second ring as before.

13.5.2 Infiltration Anaesthesia

The majority of minor surgical operations such as the excision of a small tumour or the suturing of wounds may be performed under infiltration anaesthesia. Fan-wise, infiltrate local anaesthesia (0.5%-1%) around the intended anaesthetised area, into the cutaneous and subcutaneous tissues, thereby blocking the respective sensory nerves (see Fig. 13.3). This method can be used on any body surface, e.g. head, 60 ml of 0.5%; herniatomy, 90 ml of 0.5%; Caesarean Section, 100 ml of 0.25%. The addition of adrenaline, aside from its prolonging effect, will result in a more bloodless operation field (1:200 000).

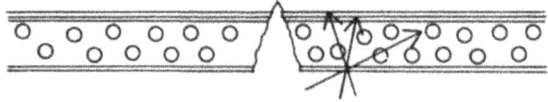

Fig. 13.3

13.5.3 Regional Anaesthesia

13.5.3.1 Digital Nerve Block

Each finger is supplied by four nerve branches:

two dorsal and two palmer, which run forward along the respective edge of the finger. The nerves of the fingers or toes are easily blocked at the base of respective digit (see Fig. 13.4).

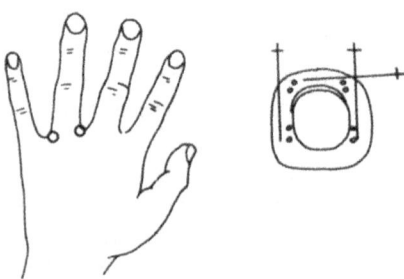

Fig. 13.4

0.5-1 ml 1%-2% local anaesthetic drug is infiltrated into the approximate course of each nerve. It is adequate to infiltrate superficially and deeply on both sides of the finger. Excessive volume of local anaesthetics should be avoided, (pressure); adrenaline should be avoided (ischaemia).

13.5.3.2 Intravenous Forearm Block

For operations on the forearm and on the hand, especially where a tourniquet is required, the IV forearm block can be used, but be sure that the blood pressure cuff is working properly. Put a needle into a good vein first (preferably in the hand), then elevate the arm, put on the cuff, secured with a bandage or plaster, and massage all the blood out. Blow up the cuff to 100 mmHg above systolic BP. Then inject 20-40 ml. 0.5% lignocaine IV. Afterwards remove the needle or close with a stopper. Analgesis will be obtained after 10 min. After the operation, there should be a time lapse of at least 30 min. Then let down the cuff for 1 s and blow up again; repeat this 3-5 times before taking off the cuff completely. The inflow of the local anaesthetic into the general circulation will thereby be slower.

13.5.3.3 Plexus Block

For operations on the forearm and hand, the plexus block can be used. The patient lies on his back, his head turned to the side. Feel the subclavian artery at the mid-point of the clavicle and mark this point (see Fig. 13.5). Stand at the head of the patient, use a 5 cm long needle and go from your marked point towards the first rib at an angle of about 80°. Before you reach the first rib, the needle will pass the plexus and the patient will feel sensation in the arm and fingers. At this point infiltrate 20 ml 2% lignocaine. *Danger: Pneumothorax.*

Fig. 13.5

In the axillary approach to the plexus block, the patient lies with the arm held at an angle of 90°. The axillary artery is palpated and the needle is inserted near the arteria (see Fig. 13.6).

The plexus lies superficially and when there is a sensation of regular pulse movement in the needle (without blood coming from the needle after aspiration),

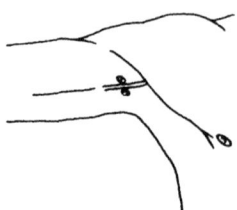

Fig. 13.6

infiltrate 20-30 ml 1% local anaesthesia. There are no contraindications for this block. *The only danger is intra-arterial injection.*

13.6 Spinal Anaesthesia

A local anaesthetic agent is introduced into the cerebrospinal fluid, which anaesthetises the spinal nerves and therefore the distal part of the body. The position and extent of the area of anaesthesia will depend upon the specific gravity of the drug. This means it depends on the rise or fall of the drug in the spinal cord space due to the position of the patient. In the anaesthetised area the sensation of pain will be abolished and profound muscular relaxation produced.

13.6.1 Anaesthetic Anatomy

When a patient lies on his back, the thoracic spine is concave upwards, the bottom of the concavity being T6, but his lumbar spine is convex upwards, the summit of the convexity being L3, the site of the lumbar puncture (see Fig. 13.7).

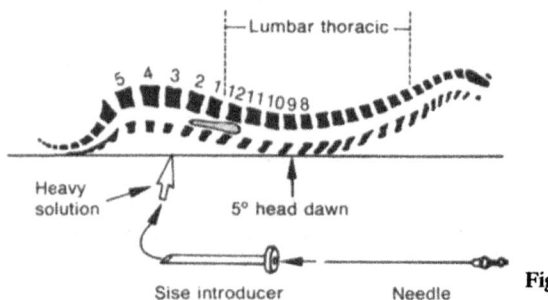

Fig. 13.7

If a heavy anaesthesia solution is introduced at this site and the patient turned flat on his back, the solution will flow down both sides of the lumbar spine, some proceeding towards the sacrum and some towards the thorax.

For an abdominal operation, the solution flowing towards the sacrum is wasted, as anaesthesia of the lower thoracic segments is required. For an abdominal operation the table is given a *slight head-down tilt*, so that the anaesthetic solution is encouraged to flow toward the thorax.

Unless the lower thoracic segments are anaesthetised in this way, the anaesthesia will fail (see Table 13.2). To ensure proper anaesthesia of the lower segments the patient is laid on his back with his knees flexed (see Fig. 13.8).

Table 13.2

Operation	Set of A. Solution
Hernia	Th 11-12
Appendices	Th 9-10
Ileus (?)	Th 9-10
Prostata	Th 12-L1
Lower Extremities	L1-L4

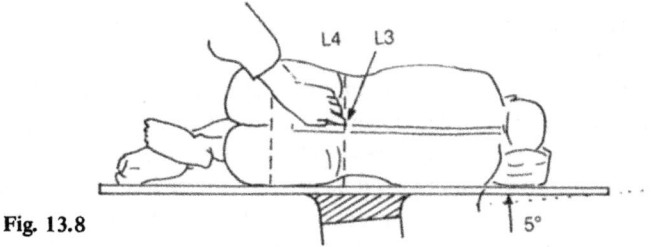

Fig. 13.8

The table is tilted $5°$ head-down *for 10 min* immediately after the anaesthetic has been given. At the end of this period the anaesthetic will have been *fixed* to the nerve roots and the patient can be turned into any position.

13.6.2 Drugs and Instruments

Heavy Nupercaine is used without adrenaline: 3 ml (15 mg) 6% solution. For the following operations the quantity of Nupercaine used is:

a) Upper abdominal operation   2 ml

b) Lower abdominal operation   1.5 ml

c) Anal-resical operation (lower spinal), cystoscopy, urethrotomy: 1 ml

The instruments required (spinal drum) are:

1 Eye towel
2 Bundles of swabs
1 Galley pot

and a small metal box containing:

2 Syringes, one 2 ml and one 5 ml to fit
2 Spinal needles with stilts
1 Fine hypodermic needle
1 Larger needle for drawing up the drug
  Ampoule files
1 Swap holder
2 Ampoules of spinal analgesia
1 Scalpel blade or size introducer

13.6.3 Method

Premedication: Neuroleptica, e.g. 0.1 mg haloperidol/kg body wt. per os 1 h
before the operation.

The patient is laid on an operating table or on a tilting trolley with the
vertebral column slightly head down. Set your spinal tray, put on gloves, but
do not open the container with the needles and syringes. Fill one galley pad
with hibitone in spirit or iodine and paint the whole of the lumbar region three
times, using a fresh swab each time. Cover with the eye towels afterwards. Sit
on a stool, so that your eye is level with the puncture site and ask a nurse to
keep the patient in the position shown in Fig. 13.8, with the back arched as
much as possible in order to open the intervertebral spaces. Choose the widest
space between two vertebrale, provided it is below L2. To identify the spines,
place one hand on the highest point of the iliac crest, which can be felt through
the sterile towels and follow a vertical line downward. This line passes over the
spine L4 or through the space between L3 and L4.

Having chosen your puncture site, make a small intradermal wheel with the
fine needle. The wheel may be made midway between two vertebrale, so that
the spinal needle can be directed straight forward or just above the lower of
the two vertebrale and the needle directed forward and upward, in the direction
of the umpilious. In either case skin in a vertical plane. If there is a size introducer, insert it through the wheel.

The introducer is a short stout needle with a stiletto (see Fig. 13.9). It reaches as far as the ligamentum flavum; the stiletto is then withdrawn and the spinal needle passes through its shaft. It prevents the fine spinal needle being bent by the ligaments and avoids any danger of sepsis or of skin particles being carried into the theca. In the absence of an introducer, the latter can be prevented by making a tiny nick in the skin with a scalpel blade and inserting the spinal needle through it. Many people, however, insert the spinal needle directly through the skin. Hold the needle by the hub and support the shaft with a swab. Never touch the point or shaft of the spinal needle with your hand.

Fig. 13.9

As the needle is felt to snap through the ligamentum flavum, withdraw the stiletto and cerebrospinal fluid will flow from the hub. If bone is encountered the needle must be withdrawn to just below the skin and inserted at a slightly different angle. If repeated difficulty is experienced, use the second spinal needle and try another interspace.

Once cerebrospinal fluid is seen to drip from the needle, attach the syringe carefully without moving the needle. Inject the required dose of anaesthesia and remove the spinal needle. Let the patient lie for 5-10 min. Turn the patient on his back, onto the sterile eye towel. Wait for another 5-10 min before putting him in the required position (see Fig. 13.10).

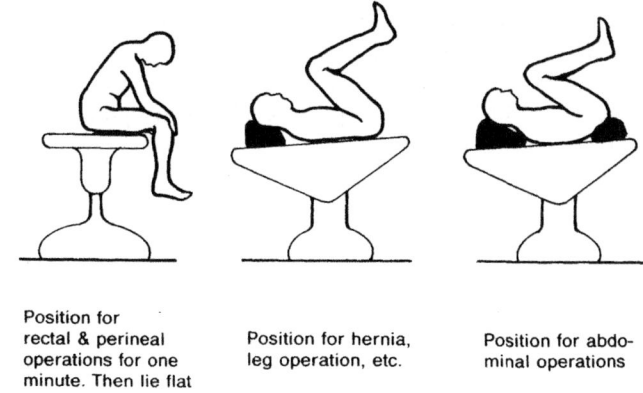

Fig. 13.10

Position for rectal & perineal operations for one minute. Then lie flat

Position for hernia, leg operation, etc.

Position for abdominal operations

Let us recall the spaces we are passing through:

skin, fat (soft resistance), ligamentum longitudinale, muscles (soft resistance), ligamentum flavum, epidural space and finally penetration of the dura (see Fig. 13.11).

117

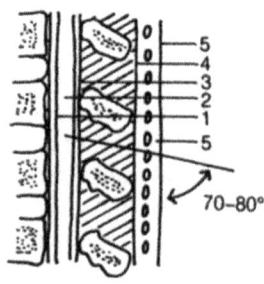

Fig. 13.11. *1* dura and intradural space, *2* epidural space, *3* ligamentum flavum, *4* ligamentum longitudinale, *5* skin

The technique of perineal anaesthesia (lower spinal) is as follows: The patient sits on the table or trolley with his feet on a stool and his neck flexed to obtain maximal flexion of the lumbar spine. The back is painted in the usual way and a sterile towel placed under the patients buttocks. 1 ml anaesthesia is injected and the patient kept sitting up for 5 min. Excellent analgesia of the perineum is obtained for the purposes of a haemorrhoidectomy, cystoscopy, etc.

13.6.4 Care and Monitoring

Obviously, the patient under spinal anaesthesia should be monitored in the same way as under general anaesthesia.

There should be a blood pressure cuff, an indwelling needle and an infusion running. Through the vasodilatating effect of the spinal anaesthesia — especially the high spinal — a fall of systolic B P below 80 mmHg is most likely, which should be corrected by a small IV dosage of a vasopressure or by a plasma-expander. It is advisable, especially after heavy premedication, to give O_2 during the operation preferably via a nasal catheter.

Post-operatively the patient must be nursed flat with a pillow and the foot of the bed raised for 6 h. For the following 6 h he must remain flat, with the bed horizontal. Then he may gradually sit up, one pillow at a time, over the next 6 h. It must be explained to him that during this time he must not sit upright for any reason. This treatment decreases the leakage of cerebrospinal fluid through the puncture in the dural and thus lowers the incidence of headaches.

13.6.5 Complications with Spinal Analgesia

Complication:	Prevention:
Headache	Use a fine spinal needle and give good post-operative care
Extradural abscess or meningitis	Absolute sterility
Paralysis (e.g. injury to cauda equina)	Do not push the needle too far beyond the dural
Cardial arrest from vasodilation and reduction of venus return	No spinal for patients with reduced circulation
Respiratory arrest	Avoid too large doses
Intubation and I.P.P.R.	

13.6.6 Indications and Contraindications

Spinal analgesia is a good anaesthesia for fit patients, where there is a definite contra-indication for general anaesthesia or no trained anaesthetist is available.
   Contraindications:

1) Sepsis anywhere on the back
2) The very ill patient, especially with reduced circulatory volume
3) Heart disease
4) Children

13.7 Epidural Anaesthesia

If this technique is performed properly, the method is safer and smoother than spinal anaesthesia.
   The only difference is that the local anaesthetic drug is introduced into the epidural space and is therefore "outside" the spinal canal. Only the extradural sensory nerves are blocked.
   The equipment required is:

1) One metal box containing
   a) Tuohy needle

b) Syringes and needles
2) Yellypot swabs and swab holder
3) Eye towels
4) Local anaesthetic: 20 ml 1%-2% with Suprarenine
5) Normal saline ampoule

The technique is similar to that of spinal anaesthesia.

The patient lies on the left side near the edge of a straight table with the knees drawn up towards the chest and the neck fully flexed.

Clean the skin and anaesthetise it and the supraspinal ligament with a thin needle. While this is taking effect, assemble the Tuohy needle and a syringe with normal saline. The Tuohy needle is then inserted through selected interspace (see Fig. 13.12). The needle is pushed slowly; the needle shaft is held with a swab with the right hand, while the left hand keeps the syringe with normal saline fixed to the hub of the needle until the ligamentum flavum is reached.

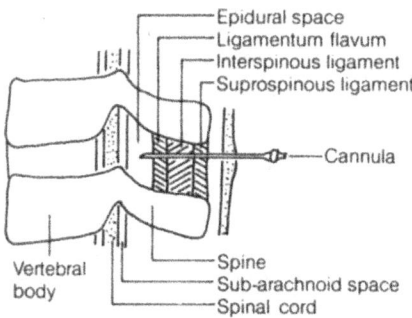

Fig. 13.12

Resistance will then be felt: slowly push through while the left hand tries to push in the normal saline. The moment the ligamentum flavum is penetrated, the normal saline can *easily* be infiltrated. Keep the needle steady!

Aspirate again, if no liquor or blood can be aspirated; if not introduce 20 ml 1%-2% local anaesthetic with Suprarenine and turn the patient gently on his back.

Anaesthesia is complete within 10-20 min and lasts for 1-2 h.

13.7.1 Complications

Dural puncture: if the dural has been injured and spinal fluid or blood cannot be aspirated, procedure has to be stopped and postponed.

Supine hypertension (vena cava compression syndrome):

This appears especially in gravid uterus, restricting venous return of blood to the heart by pressing backwards on the inferior vena cava. Symptoms include pallor, ringing in the ears, faintness and nausea. Treatment is simple: turn the patient onto herside, preferably the left side.

Chapter 14
Management of Emergency Situations

14.1 Cardiac Arrest

The best definition of cardiac arrest I ever came across is that given by Safar who wrote:

"Cardiac arrest is the clinical picture of cessation of circulation in a patient who was not expected to die at that time." The phrase "a patient who was not expected to die at that time" indicates the need for reanimation.

The diagnosis of cardiac arrest is simple (see Fig. 14.1).

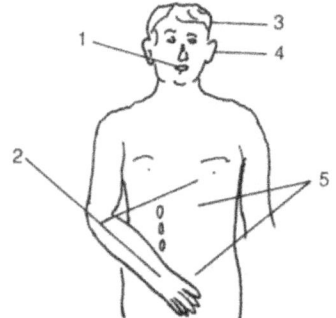

Fig. 14.1. *1* no spontaneous respiration, *2* no pulse, *3* unconsciousness, *4* dilated pupils, *5* loss of natural colour

There are five cardiac symptoms:

1) No spontaneous respiration
2) No pulse
3) Unconsciousness (not applicable during general anaesthesia)
4) Loss of natural colour
5) Dilated pupils

Usually, the patient becomes unconscious 6 s after circular breakdown, breathing stops after 15 s (the heart sometimes still "moves" for a couple of seconds) and the pupils dilate after 1 min. If the above five symptoms are present in a patient, you may be sure of cardiac insufficiency or cardiac arrest.

The success of reanimation depends on quick action. This means immediate artificial oxygenation and artificial circulation. No time should be wasted looking for the reasons for the cardiac arrest. More important at that moment is artificial ventilation and circulation, following the A.B.C. rule:

A) Airway opened
B) Breathing restored
C) Circulation restored

A) Firstly, clear the *airway* with a sucker or if this is not available, with a gauze and your finger (see Fig. 14.2). You must be absolutely sure that the air passage is free from any mechanical blockage.

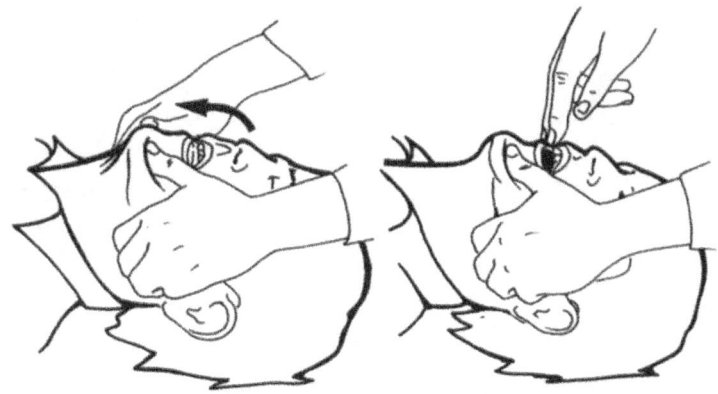

Fig. 14.2

B) *Restore breathing:* in the case of hyperventilation, mouth to mouth breathing oxygenates the blood sufficiently (see Fig. 14.3). Advantages of the mouth to mouth breathing method: it can be applied at once without looking for instruments: the blockage of the airway is shown immediately and the expansion of the thorax can be observed.

Optimal ventilation is achieved by endotracheal intubation, and ideally, I.P.P.V. (see Fig. 14.4). If you are not familiar with intubation, time should not be wasted waiting for the instrument and trying to intubate.

Do not waste time! Ventilate by all means and by any means!

C) Restore circulation with external heart massage (first introduced in 1960 by Rouwenhoven).

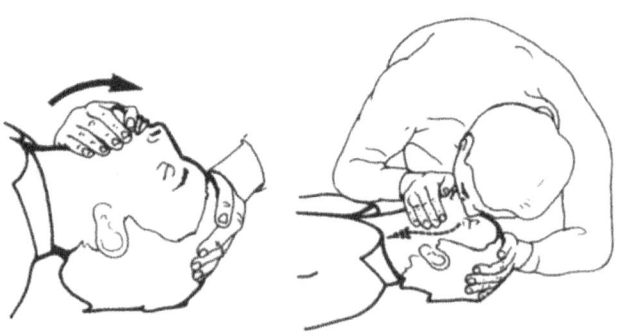

Fig. 14.3. Right position for mouth to mouth breathing

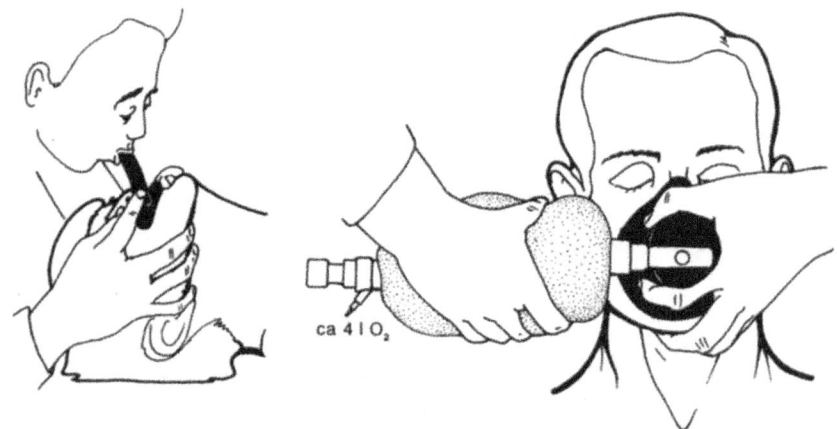

ca 4 l O_2

Fig. 14.4. Besides there are instruments to be used instead of the mouth to mouth breathing method, e.g. Safar tube, breathing bag

To avoid any damage the external heart massage should be applied in the following way:

1) The patient should lie on his back on a hard board or on the floor, if possible with legs up (modified shock position).
2) Put the palm of one of your hands on the last third of the sternum and assisting with the other hand rhythmically push at least 2 inches down (see Fig. 14.5).

By this process the heart will be pressed between the sternum and the spine, the thorax acting like a spring, expanding the heart during the resting phase. The result will be a rhythmic inflow and outflow of blood in the heart.

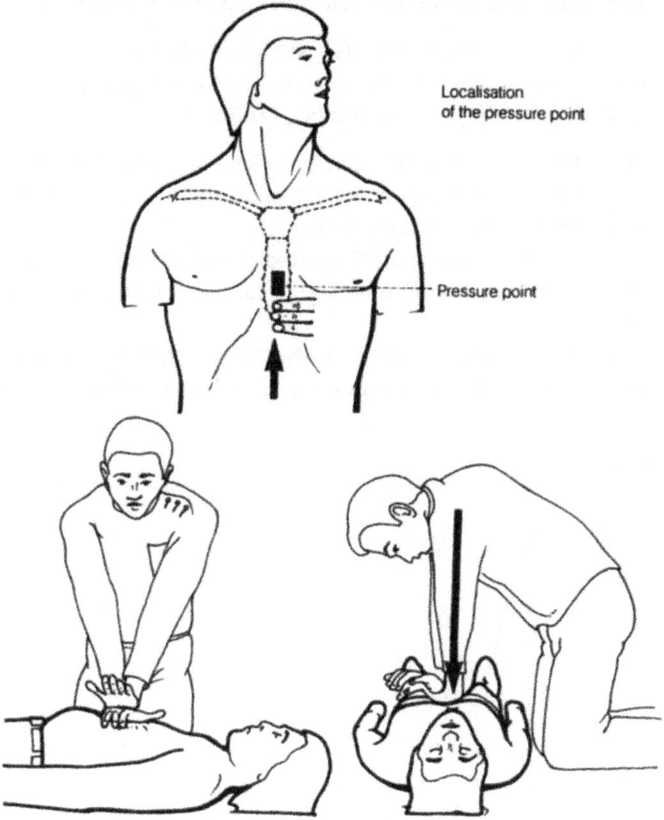

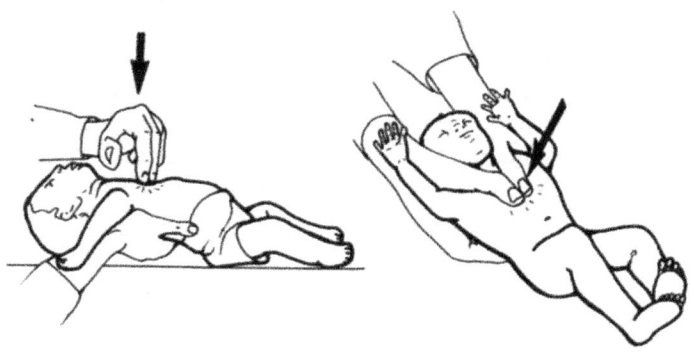

Fig. 14.5

The procedure of heart massage in children differs according to age. With the neonatal, take the baby's chest between two fingers and thumb and press in and out (Fig. 14.6).

Fig. 14.6

For older children use only one hand instead of two as described for adults.

Reanimation can be performed by one person, but it is much easier to having two people working: one on heart massage and the other on artificial breathing. The rhythm should be as follows:

Five times heart massage, once or twice breathing. This process should be repeated at least 12 times per min, which means at least 60 heart massages per min. With children double this number.

Soon after starting artificial respiration, give Alupent or adrenaline 0.5-1.0 ml intracardial (if there is complete cardiac arrest), otherwise it should be given IV.

Research in the last few years has shown that cardiac arrest gives an extreme metabolic and respiratory acidosis after 1 min with pH under 7.1.

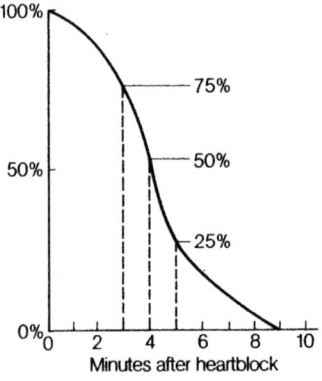

Fig. 14.7. Chance of success

This is clearly not an ideal condition for recovery from cardiac arrest. Therefore it is important to give sodium bicarbonate ($NaHCO_3$); for every minute of cardiac arrest 50 mg $NaHCO_3$. Experience has shown that 150 ml 8.4% sodium bicarbonate solution is sufficient to start with. After this give 10 ml 10% solution calcium chloride, followed by an IV application of plasmaexpander. The administration of an IV injection will cause some difficulties since often the peripherial vessels have collapsed. However, in such a case, one should not hesitate to use the vena anonyma or vena jugularis. Its volume is always open and with practice this is not difficult to achieve (see Fig. 14.8).

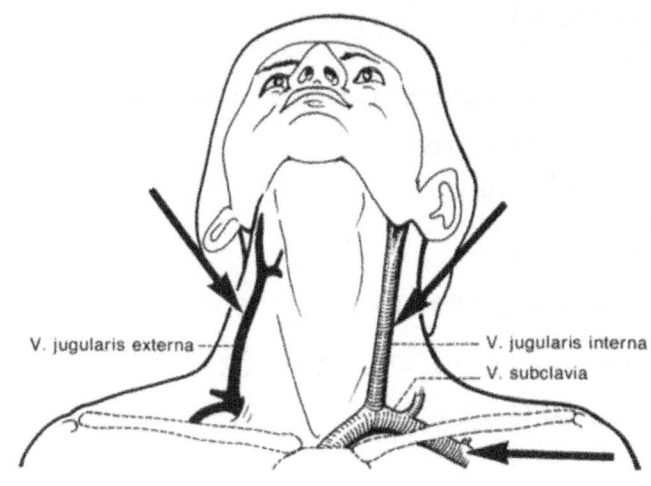

V. jugularis externa

V. jugularis interna

V. subclavia

Fig. 14.8

14.1.1 Summary

1) Diagnosis:
    a) No breathing
    b) No pulse
    c) Unconscious
    d) Dilated pupils
2) Action
    a) Put patient on hard board or floor
    b) Clear airway and start ventilation *by any means*
    c) Look for help
    d) Start with external heart massage
    e) Drugs: Alupent or adrenaline; calcium chloride; plasma-expander
    f) 150 ml 8.3% solution sodium bicarbonate

14.2 Shock

There are three different major reasons for shock:

1) *Haemorrhagic shock:*

   Lack of volume

2) *Cardiac shock:*

   Weakening of the pump

3) *Maximal dilatation of vascular system*

   Anaphylactic shock
   Toxic shock

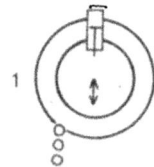

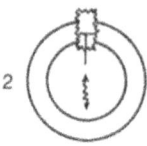

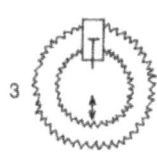

Signs and Symptoms

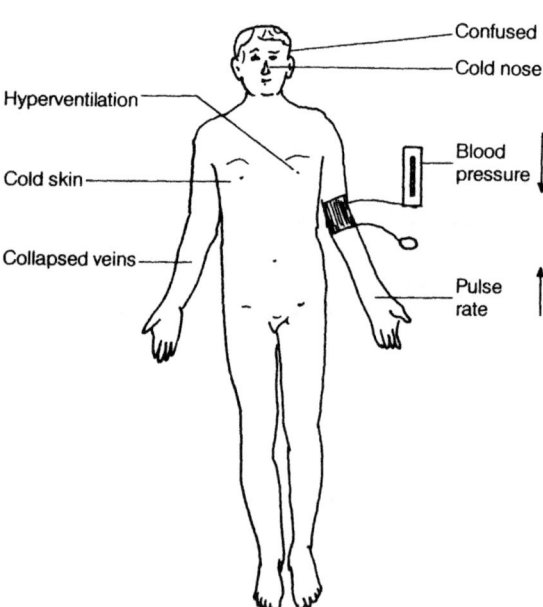

a) Normal functions

The total quantity of blood in the human body amounts to 8%-9% of the body weight, e.g. a man weighing 70 kg would have 6.5 litres of blood.

b) Irregular functions

Shock due to fluid loss

A reduction of the blood circulating in the body can be caused by visible haemorrhages and also by haemorrhages in body cavities and in tissues.

Furthermore, loss of body fluid, e.g. in the case of burns, diarrhoea and vomiting leads not only to a reduction of the circulatory blood volume but also to a "thickening (condensation) of blood" (less liquid, more blood cells). In both cases an insufficient volume of blood causes a disturbance of the blood distribution. Moreover, transportation of blood is aggravated because it is not able to flow properly when thicker. As a protection mechanism (emergency reaction) a centralisation of the circulation is started, i.e. the vessels become tighter with a corresponding decrease in blood circulation, mainly in the skin and skeletal muscles, in order to supply vital organs such as the heart, lung and brain with enough blood.

In other words: the reduced blood volume causes a reduction of the circulation and a reduction of the area supplied. At the same time the heart is stimulated (sympathicus), in order to pump across a tachycardia the reduced blood quantity more quickly through the system. Only in this way can the O_2 requirement of life-essential organs be secured in the reduced circulation.

The consequence is the development of an acute decrease (blood) circulation of the tissues with increasing lack of oxygen (oxygen deficiency) of the individual cells. According to the extent of the hypoxia, reversible damage occurs first and irreversible damage later.

Indication

Visible signs of shock:

Pallidness (minor circulation of the periphery).
Reduced filling of veins/venous collapse (centralisation).
Hyperthermia (peripheral minor blood circulation and disorder of the vegetative nervous system).
Unusual psychic behaviour, restlessness or rigidity (disorder) of the nervous and (autonomic) vegetative nervous system.

Tangible signs of shock:

Fast and shallow pulse (100-140).
Slightly suppressible pulse (indirect sign for low blood pressure).
Cold skin (under circulation of periphery).
Circulation delay in the nail bed (matrix), reduced circulation of the skin (dermal) capillaries, centralisation.
Cold sweat (disorder of the vegetative nervous system).

Measurable signs of shock:

Arterial blood pressure (decline of the systolic blood pressure, mainly below 100 mmHg).
Shock index: proportion (relation) pulse rate systolic blood pressure.

Normal:

Pulse 60, systolic blood pressure 120
Index $\frac{60}{120} = 0.5$
In shock situations:

a) pulse 100, systolic blood pressure 100

Index $\frac{100}{100} = 1.0$

b) pulse 120, systolic blood pressure 80

Index $\frac{120}{80} = 1.5$

Central Venous Pressure (CVP):
Normal: pressure between 3 to 6 cm water column.

In shock situation below zero, suction!
(A rough estimate is made after inserting a catheter in the vena cava by removing the infusion system and *holding the drip at chest level.*)

Practical Advice

With a pulse and a blood pressure of about 100 always check for shock, take the corresponding emergency aid measures and check the circulation system at short intervals in order to be able to diagnose a recovery or a deterioration.

The following is fundamental:

The higher the pulse rate is above 100, the lower the blood pressure under 100, the more dangerous the shock is. The 100/100 rule is used as a guide. Particularly with young adolescent patients the tachycardia is often the most impressive sign of shock, the decline in blood pressure follows relatively late but then often very dramatically.

Acute Volume Overload

Particularly in emergency cases, in the treatment of shock it can come to a unjustified supply of blood volume substitutes in the stress of the situation, as the rise in the frequency of the pulse rate and the minor circulation of the skin often remain stable for the time being – even after sufficient volume supply.

Blood pressure rises, however, when the haemorrhages could be staunched. Therefore, it is also necessary to make blood pressure controls more often during the volume supply.

Indications

Visible indications: increased filling of veins near the heart most clearly visible on vena jugularis externa.

Estimation of CVP, vein pressure over 14 cm H_2O (with central venous catheter).

A possible development of a pulmonary oedema as a sign of a heavy volume load mainly of the left part of the heart.

14.3 Poisoning

Management of Parathion Poisoning

Signs and Symptoms	Elimination and Block in Action of Toxin	Maintenance of Respiratory	Vital Body functions Cardio and Metabolic	Remarks
I. *Mental Stage* Semiconsciousness Respiration: Ø Card: bradycardia Hypotony Reflexes: ✓ Muscle twisting Ø	Stomach washout Atropine up to 1 mg hourly Tachycardia – 140 Forced diuresis Lasix and infusion	1. Clean airway 2. Observation	Infusion: N.S. and dextrose 1 2 up to 6 l Lasix – 1000 ml inf. 20 mg	I.C.U. Careful In and output Psychological help Haloperidol 0.5 x 3
II. and III. 1 Ental Stage Unconsciousness *Respiratory:* ↓ *C: – Shock* ✓ *Bradycardia* ✓ Reflexes Ø	Stomach washout? Atropine 20-30 min 0.6 mg (0.01 mg/kg) Tachycardia – 140 per min. Forced diuresis	1. airway obst. 2. lung oedema 3. paralysation – C.R.G. Clear airway Intubation – Ambubag – no C.N. stimulant	→ ← →	Convulsions Valium 5 mg i.v. every 2-3 hours I.C.U. Urine output control
IV. *Mental Stage* Coma ✓ Convulsions ✓ Respiratory: ↓↓	Atropine 0.6 mg every 15 min. I.v.	Intubation Ambubag	Plasma expander Infusion 1-2	"

C: – bradycardia↓

Reflexes ∅

Lasix HCO$_3$ 100 ml

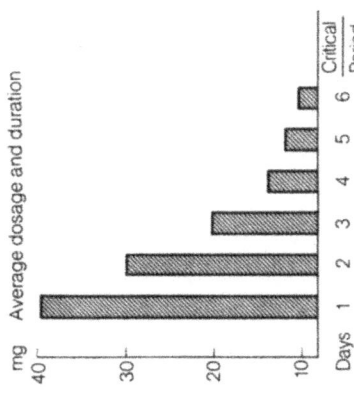

mg   Average dosage and duration

Days 1 2 3 4 5 6   Critical
                        Period

Summary

1. Maintenance of the vital body functions
2. Atropinisation
3. Elimination of not yet absorbed toxins
4. Forced diuresis

133

Chapter 15
Fluids and Electrolytes

It is important to the anaesthetist that there is proper pre-, intra- and post-anaesthetic water and electrolyte management. "There are more people dying of thirst in bed than in the desert". On average, 60% of the human body consists of water divided as follows:

1) Intracellular
2) Extracellular
   a) Interstitial
   b) Intravessel
   c) Transcellular
(see Fig. 15.1 and Tables 15.1 and 15.2)

Furthermore, the body produces 7-8 litres of fluid per day, which, however, is mostly reabsorbed.

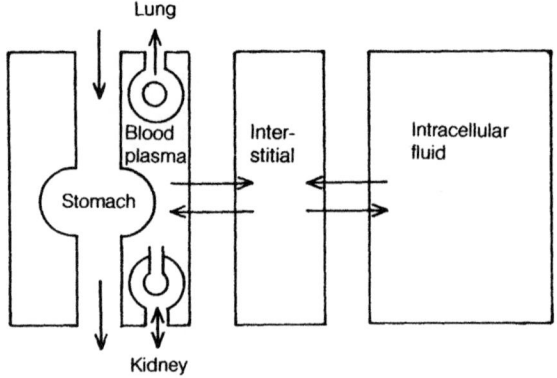

Fig. 15.1

Table 15.1. Composition of the electrolyte

in mVal	Plasma	Interstitial	Intracellular
Na^+	136-142	140	10-12
Cl^-	103	103-115	10- 2
K^+	4.3	4-5	150-145
HCO_3	25	24-30	10-12
Ca^{++}	5	4	

Table 15.2

	Urine	Sweat	Stomach fluid	Pancreas
Na^+	100-180	5	60	110-150
Cl^-	100-160	45	100 !!	4-5
K^+	50-100	10	8-10	50-80
HCO_3	6	–	–	120
TOT.AM.	1500 ml –	– 500 ml –	2000 ml –	ca. 600 ml

15.1 Acidosis and Alkalosis

Acids are substances which can release H^+ ions.
Alkali are substances which can receive H^+ ions.
The pH factor demonstrates whether a fluid is acidic or alkaline.
The physiological point is pH 7.4 (see Fig. 15.2).

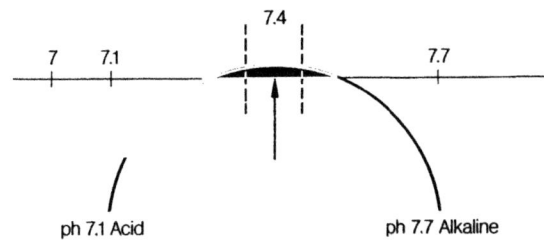

Fig. 15.2

For maintenance of a normal acid and alkaline balance the body has different possibilities:

a) The lungs can excrete CO_2
b) The kidneys can excrete HCO_3
c) The puffer substances in the blood — $NaHCO_3$
   (substances which are able to "fix" H ions)

The pH is maintained because the relative amounts of $NaHCO_3$ and CO_2 are kept constant by the compensating activity of the lungs and kidneys.

Acidosis and alkalosis result from respiratory or metabolic disturbances, which may overthrow the physiological balance in four possible ways (see Table 15.3).

1) *Respiratory Acidosis:* Hypoventilation and increase of CO_2, e.g. after anaesthesia, pneumonia, emphysema, or abdominal distension.
2) *Metabolic acidosis:* Increase of organic acid substance (H-ions), e.g. in diabetes, kidney failure, C.C.F., shock-impaired peripheral circulation and cardiac arrest. The buffer system in the blood (bicarbonate) can no longer cope and consequently these patients need $NaHCO_3$.
3) *Respiratory alkalosis:* Hyperventilation and decrease of CO_2, e.g. in tetany and hysteria.
4) *Metabolic alkalosis:* To free substitute of bicarbonate or long-standing vomiting (loss of chlorine).

Input

Total daily maintenance fluid amount

B W	ml/kg B W	Calories/24 h
3	68	170
5	77	320
7	82	480
9	80	600
11	80	720
13	72 !	780
15	68	850
17	66	940
19	63	1000
21	61	1060
25	57	1180
29	54	1300

Over 20 kg B W = 1500 ml + 25 ml for each kg over 20 kg

Table 15.3

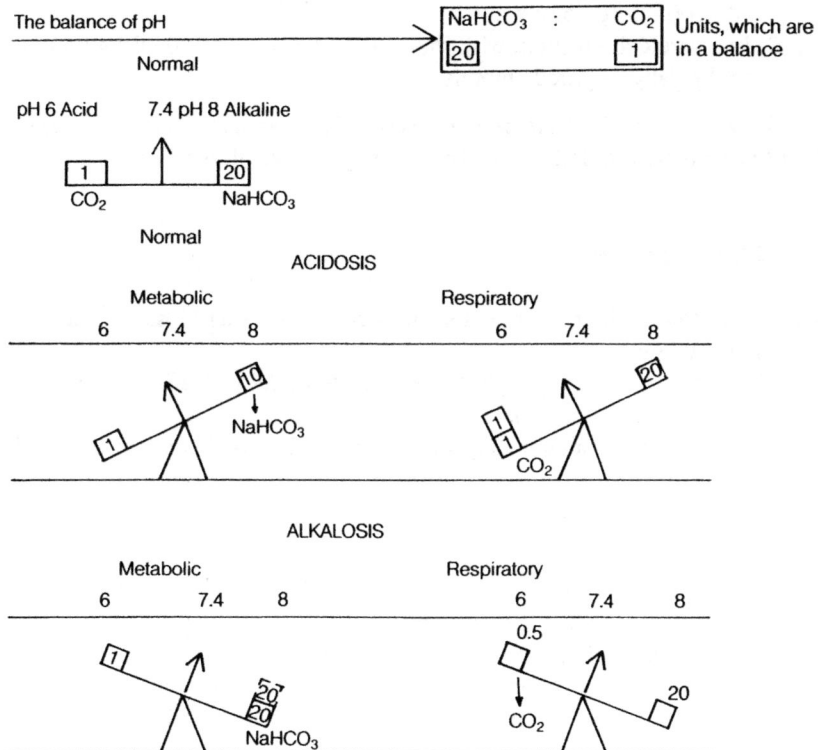

15.2 Electrolytes

2 Na^+ mVal/kg body wt. but no more than 15 mg Na^+ mVal/kg/body wt./24 h

2 Cl^- mVal/kg body wt. but no more than 15 mg Cl^- mVal/kg/body wt./24 h

1 K^+ mVal/kg body wt. but no more than 3 mg K^+ mVal/kg body wt./24 h

(K^+ is usually not given in the first 24 h post-operatively)

15.2.1 Pre-Operative

In the case of pre-operative dehydration, estimate the stage:

1) In mild dehydration that is just perceptible add 50 ml/kg body wt.
2) In moderate dehydration, with signs of dehydration but no shock, add 100 ml/kg body wt.
3) In severe dehydration, with shock and apathy, add 150 ml/kg body wt. to the daily required amount.

Always try to rehydrate before anaesthesia. It is usually safe to replace half the estimated deficit in 2 h. The rest is given over 4, 6 and 8 h.

15.2.2 Intra-Operative

Remember that with an open abdomen or chest the patient loses, unseen, 300 ml every hour.

Give babies one-half strength Ringer lactate or 0.45% NaCl (infused at a rate of 10 ml/kg body wt./h).

Give children and adults Ringer lactate or 0.45% NaCl at a rate of 6 ml/kg body wt./h.

15.2.2.1 Blood Transfusion

A blood loss of 10% of the blood volume causes little visible change in the circulation of a fit patient. Venous constriction maintains a normal venous return and cardiac output, except where this mechanism is interrupted by drugs. Greater losses of blood result in a fall of venous pressure and cardiac output, but blood pressure may be maintained at normal level by intense arterial constriction until much greater losses have occurred.

The hypotensive patient may have lost 50% of his blood!

The pulse rate, venous filling, skin colour and temperature, urine flow together with P.C.V. and Hgb., are the best guides for estimating the blood loss.

When the blood loss exceeds 15%-20% of the blood volume, replacement of some of the loss by blood transfusion is desirable. The blood volume is approximately 80 ml/kg body wt. Ringer lactate solution is the best initial treatment in the shock patient as it reduces blood viscosity and improves tissue perfusion. While the Ringer lactate solution is being given, blood can be crossmatched.

Adequate replacement should result in the reversal of the signs of blood loss. The circulatory stability (B P and pulse) together with an adequate urine output is a useful guide to the circulatory filling.

Remember: Transfusion blood contains citrate (anti-coagulant). Rapid infusion can result in citrate intoxication, so give with each second bottle of blood, 1 g calcium gluconate through a separate IV needle.

15.2.3 Post-Operative

The patient will need the normal daily requirements for the next 24 h, plus any anticipated losses.

0.18% NaCl + 5% glucose is a suitable fluid solution. Patients with peritonitis need more fluid and are short of colloids, so the clinical picture has to be guide. In the first 24 h after operation, K^+ is not normally given.

15.2.3.1 Acidosis

Patients with poor peripheral circulation or a history of this will produce lactic acid as a result of anaerobic metabolism. Patients with poor renal function will not be able to excrete a normal acid load. The severely dehydrated patient has both problems and therefore is usually acidotic.

Acidosis depresses the heart and circulation.

Give 2 mg $NaHCO_3$/kg body wt. (Sodium bicarbonate helps to combat metabolic acidosis and to improve the patient's general condition.) 8.4% $NaHCO_3$ solution contains 1 mval/ml.

In addition to the post-operative IV fluid and maintenance of calories a rectal drip can be given overnight.

It is very cheap and can be easily prepared in a solution of 50g dextrose, 10g alcohol and 500 ml water, to be given rectally at a rate of not more than 16 drops/min.

Chapter 16

Intensive Care Unit (I.C.U.)

The anaesthetist is responsible for the patient for up to 36 h post-anaesthesia. Post-operative conditions of the patient can change and therefore need continuous and careful observation. Intensive care means extensive and continual careful observation and treatment of patients who suffer from *insufficient functioning* of one or more of the following systems:

1) Respiratory system
2) Circulatory system
3) Metabolic system

The danger of failure of any of the above mentioned systems is a clear indication for a patient to be admitted into the I.C.U. The patient should, however, be returned to his respective department as soon as the major threat has passed. This means a centralisation of patients needing intensive care, but not necessarily a unit of surgical patients only, especially as in smaller hospitals a concentration of all the more seriously ill patients is advisable.

The lay-out of an I.C.U. is a compromise between the present economical, technical and manpower situation and the continuous drive towards improvement and further development. It is therefore a beginning which has to be improved on continually, according to the situation. The functioning of an intensive care unit requires trained personnel, special establishment and equipment.

16.1 Trained Personnel

One of the important factors of an I.C.U. is the nursing care and much of the success depends on the co-operation of the nursing staff. The duties of the nurses in an I.C.U. are divided between two main objects: to give proper and responsible *nursing care* and to maintain proper *management* of the unit. This includes proper maintenance of the equipment (checking of oxygen suction, pump, etc.).

It is the responsibility of the staff nurse to create a co-operative team spirit among the staff, besides keeping the unit up to the maximum standard. One day every week all technical equipment must be checked and the necessary repairs done. The main responsibility of the staff nurse is the *organisation* and the *management* of the daily routine.

In the average schedule every staff member works 5 days and has 2 off-days (see Table 16.1).

Table 16.1. The functioning of an Intensive Care Unit, continued. Working hours in day time can be divided as follows

Group	Time	Mo	Tu	We	Th	Fr	Sa	Su
	8-11		off					
I.	12- 5		duty					
	8-12							
II.	2- 6				off			
	8-1							
III.	3-6						off	

IV. Staff nurse – takes off at convenience

V. Night duty 6 p.m. – 8 a.m. (the overtime is compensated by night duty offs.)

5 working days x 8 h/day means 40 working h/week.

On night duty there should be two nurses or aides who alternate one week night duty and one week off, in rotation with the other staff.

There must always be someone present who is responsible for the unit, with proper handing-over of the unit between duties. The day and night handing-over should be done by a registered nurse.

The total staff number should be fairly high: one nurse per two patients during the day and one nurse per eight patients at night. This personnel, however, could in part be released from other departments, since all the patients who need special care and observation would be in the I.C.U.

The overall responsibility of daily organisation should be in the hands of the nursing officer in charge of the unit. This includes admission and discharge of patients in co-operation with the medical officer.

The medical responsibility lies in the hands of the particular medical officer.

16.2 Special Establishment

The bed capacity should be 4% of the total beds in the hospital. The unit should be near to the theatre and cut-off from the normal route of visitors. The arrangement of beds should give 9 m^2 per bed. Together with the bathrooms, store rooms, toilets, etc. there should be 21 m^2 per bed. The beds should be arranged to allow observation of each one (see Fig. 16.1).

It is important to adhere to the given square meterage because of the necessity of having much working space and for the possible addition of technical equipment.

There is no necessity for the separation of males and females; curtains or screens provide the necessary privacy. There should be, however, strict separation between septic and aseptic patients, as shown in the plan. Generally, visitors or helpers should not be admitted, except with the permission of the officer in charge of the unit.

If visitors are admitted, they must wear special gowns provided by the hospital.

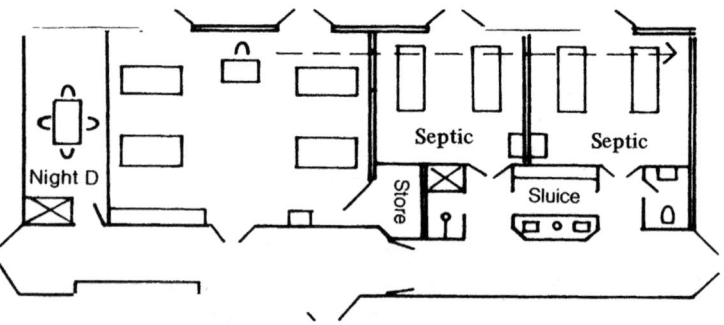

Fig. 16.1

16.3 Equipment

The following is a list of equipment which is *absolutely necessary*, easy to maintain and relatively cheap:

1) One oxygen unit *for each side* (septic and aseptic)
2) One suction machine for each side (foot operated)
3) Transportable adjustable light for each room (locally made)

4) BP equipment and stethoscope for each room
5) At least two measuring glasses for each side, two urinometers, etc.
6) One steam inhaler for each side
7) Beds with hard boards and head- and leg-elevators
8) A portable trolley adjustable to each bed
9) Three weed bags for each bed with washable covers
10) Three hot water bottles for the whole unit
11) One scale

The most practical piece of equipment is an emergency trolley (made locally from wood: 50 x 100 x 75 cm, see Fig. 16.2) which should comprise the following:

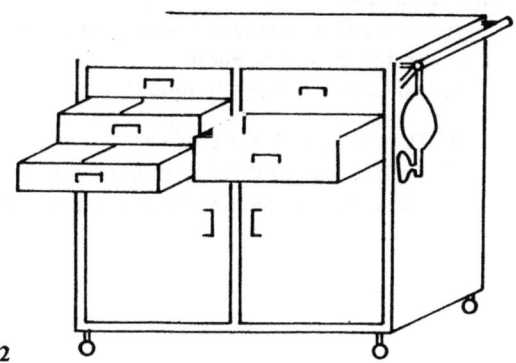

Fig. 16.2

The first four drawers contain medicine (ampoules), listed infusion and sets (Ringer, Manite, Plasma, Na HCO$_3$, etc.). The fifth and sixth drawers hold technical equipment:

a) Airways (Guedel, nasal tubes)
b) Feeding tubes
c) Torch
d) Measuring glass
e) BP apparatus and stethoscope
f) Pleura needle
g) Infusion sets for children (scalp vein set)
h) Two dressing packs
i) Suction tubes
j) Veno-pressure set
k) Observation cards

The seventh drawer contains emergency sets:

a) Cut down
b) Catheter bag
c) Hand suction machine
d) Intubation bag
e) Emergency bag
f) Ambubag (artificial respiration bag)

For the precise control of each patient we use the Machame Observation Card (see Fig. 16.3), where, as far as possible, the therapy is written down for the next 24 h. The nursing sister has to go at least once every hour to each bed to check what medication or other procedure has to be carried out. There is also a monitoring guide in each room with the seven points which have to be checked hourly.

Every medical aide who has worked in a functional I.C.U. knows the value of such a unit at any hospital.

It will work successfully only if:

1) The unit is not overcrowded
2) The staff know its responsibilities, is well trained and dedicated
3) The necessary technical equipment is available

Monitoring of Seriously Ill Patients

1. General Impression

a) *Conscious* — quiet
b) *Unconscious* — *danger*

restless – danger – — bleeding
— check B P – doctor

1. General Impression

Feeding – infusion-stomach tube
bed sores – change position and
airway – clear airway – pr.
pneumonia

2. Airway

Respiration
14–20 min.

quick resp.
bleeding B P
↓
danger – doctor
↑
— forced resp.
↓
— clear airway
↓
→ sucker

3. Circulation

4. Feeding + infusion

Check the right infusion
(feeding) speed, no swelling -input

5. Urine output and drainage

Urine 30 ml/hour
check amount? specific gravity
record sugar, albumin, etc.

6. Temperature

Child above 39° C (tepid sponge – doctor –)

3. Circulation

High B P — B P — Pulse

200/140

Doctor
↓
low B P
↓
Danger
↓
Bleeding – infusion
Pulse
↓
Doctor

100 and age

70–100 min.

Slow pulse – quick pulse

Head injury — *Danger – shock*
↓   ↓
Doctor   B P infusion
                    ↓
                Doctor

7. Observation chart

What has to be done according
to the chart – time – record –

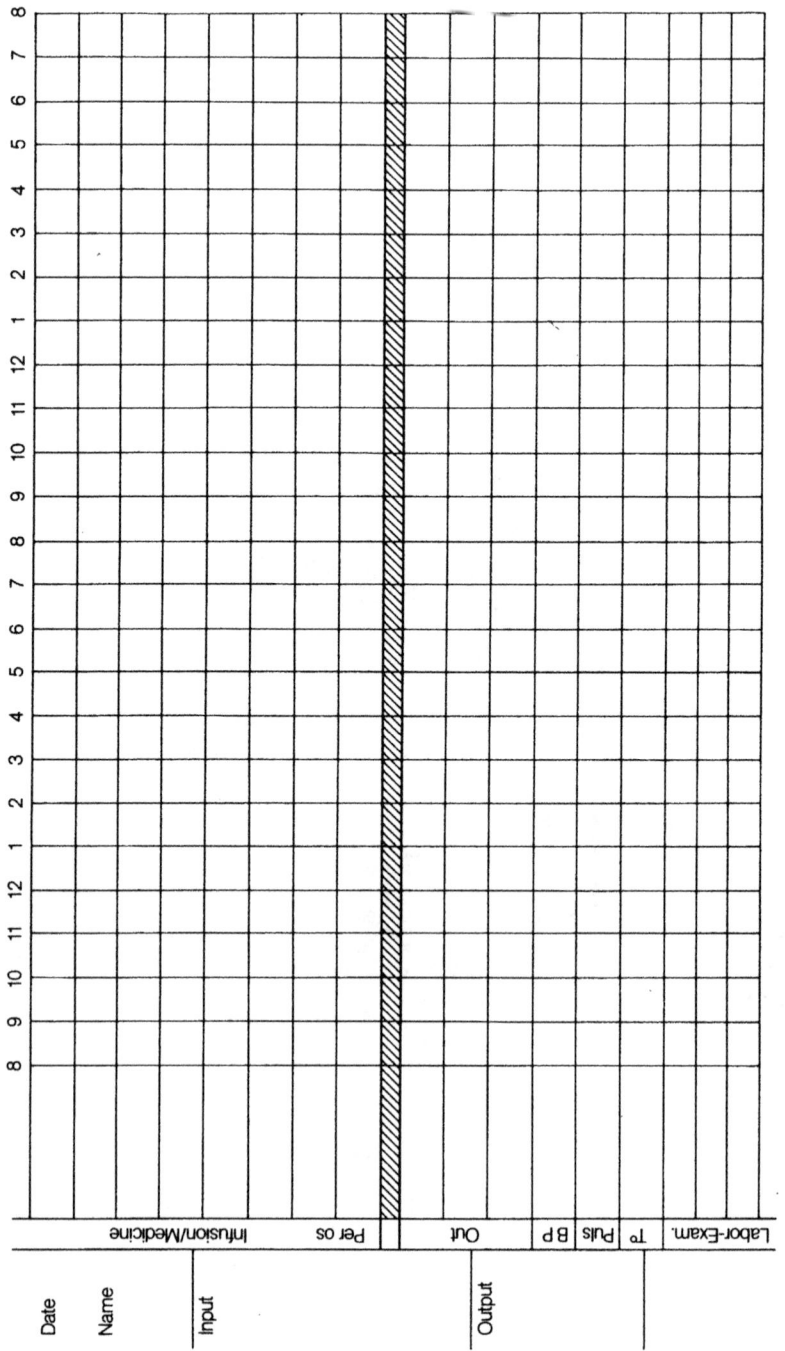

Fig. 16.3

146

Chapter 17
Fear and Confidence

Psychological preparation of a patient for anaesthesia and surgery is vital!

Professor Frey of Mainz University suggests, in an article on the factor of fear as an influence on a patient before anaesthesia and surgery, how an anaesthetist can prepare a patient in a positive way for his operation.

It would seem that fear is universal for people facing anaesthesia and surgery; the causes of fear, however, are somewhat different in technically advanced countries from those in developing countries.

In the former, mass media, (television, radio, the press, etc.,) greatly influence the patient, either positively or negatively, in his approach towards hospitalisation. He is familiar with the atmosphere of a hospital, he has seen, or read about, oxygen-cylinders, lifts and other normal technical equipment found in the hospital and he is also familiar with the basic procedure in an operating theatre.

The situation is entirely different in developing countries, for instance, Tanzania, where most people are nearer to the soil than to the wheel, living in closer contact with nature than with technology. They do not get worried about the possibility of an empty oxygen tank, unclean syringes or an uncomfortable anaesthetic mask, as these things are beyond their personal experience; they are, however, somewhat afraid for four main reasons:

1. The patient finds himself in a *strange new situation* and *separated from his family.* More than 50% of the patients that enter the hospital have already consulted their "local doctor". The reason is not a financial one, as the patient invariably pays more to the local doctor than he would have to pay at the hospital. Payments to the local doctor extend over periods of up to as many as five years. The reason for consulting the local doctor is the patient's confidence in him, because the treatment given is "traditional". The medicines used are familiar herbs, roots, skins or "charms", etc., whose imaginative healing powers are known.
The main reason may possibly be that the local doctor is nearby and consulting him does not separate the patient from his home, his family and his

own normal daily surroundings and put him in a new and strange situation. The hospital and the strange sight of the operating theatre and its attendants with all its alarming equipment, causes considerable anxiety and fear in the patient; he becomes more suspicious the more sophisticated the hospital.

2. He is anxious about *losing his independence.* At first sight, the patient's dependence upon others does not seem to bother him much, but when he comes to consider it more in detail, it turns out to be a deeply important factor. Who likes to surrender his whole existence to some unknown person and completely depend on him for help? This discomfort is likely to be more important to men than it is to women: it contradicts social custom for a man to depend for help or even to take orders from a female nurse.

3. The patient always has a *fear of death* to some degree. From previous experiences in the family and with neighbours, the patient accepts the existence of death and also of pain, and provided there is a good chance of recovery, he does not worry much about pain and discomfort. Fear of a technical failure during an operation does not occur to him as it does in patients in developed countries, but fear associated with possible death is always present, especially as the procedures of an operation are beyond his imagination.

4. The *fear of becoming handicapped* after the operation originates from the social and economic situation in Tanzania. In Kiswahili the *maskini* or the really deprived are the handicapped and the crippled who cannot support themselves and have to depend on others for survival. Consequently, when a patient is told, for instance, that part of his stomach is to be removed because of an ulcer, he immediately associates this with the idea that he will not be able to eat anymore, so that he will lose strength and will not be able to cultivate his soil to produce food for his own living and that of his family. In other words, the patient thinks that the operation is going to destroy him and that he will end up a *maskini.*

Yet, in spite of all these fears, there are several reasons why a patient will go to the hospital and will agree to have an operation under anaesthesia.

a) Man always has the *disposition to get better!* Under all circumstances there is a strong will to be cured and to become a capable member of his society again. Since the government and the churches have provided hospitals as "body repair shops", the patient will try these places, though often as the last resort and often too late.

b) Confidence in a particular hospital or doctor is usually gained by reputation: perhaps a patient has heard from neighbours or friends that a cer-

tain hospital or doctor is good and he therefore can get reliable help from
him.

c) Fatalism or faith also play their part. To the patient his illness seems something beyond his control, just like many other phenomena of his experience, such as crop failure, lack of rain or death. God had decided it to be
that way, so there is very little he can do about it.

We use a scale to demonstrate these points (see Fig. 17.1).

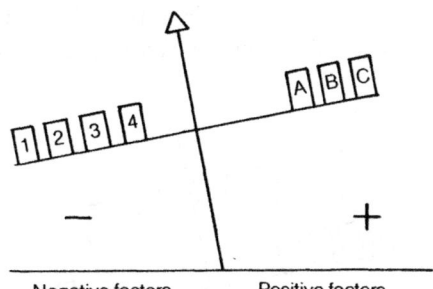

Fig. 17.1   Negative factors   Positive factors

On one side the negative factors: the patients fears and anxieties, and on the
other side the positive factors: the reasons why he will go to hospital.

What can be done to reduce the negative factors and to build up a strong
positive attitude towards the hospital? I see a possibility of *utilising the positive factors* to remove fear and worries and to use his *fatalism* and his *faith*
to build up confidence in the hospital, the staff and all the procedures involved.

A patient who is resigned to his fate does not fear death since whatever
has been decided will happen, and faith faces death in acceptance of God's
will and decision. The patient sees his illness as something beyond his control
and which he himself and even his local doctor are unable and incapable of
dealing with, so he goes to the hospital resigned to his fate.

It is up to us now to build up his confidence, as this is another important
factor. A patient who has confidence is not confused by a strange situation;
he is inclined to allow himself to become dependent because he is convinced
that the hospital, its facilities and the personnel involved are likely to help him
and will not make him a cripple or a *maskini.* As soon as he has confidence in
someone he will feel safe and at home. It is necessary to increase the patient's
confidence as much as possible:

1) Take time to see the patient before he is anaesthetised.
2) Listen to his complaints.

149

3) Explain what will happen to him. Tell him that *you* will take care of him when he sleeps and when he is unable to help himself. If he feels pain, explain to him that he will be given medicine to make him comfortable. Assure him that he will not feel any pain during the operation and that when he wakes up it will all be over. In the meantime, *you will be there for his sole benefit.*
4) Relax him by talking with him about his family or something else of personal interest to him.

In this way as shown in Fig. 17.2 it is possible to diminish fear and discomfort and to build up confidence by using fatalism.

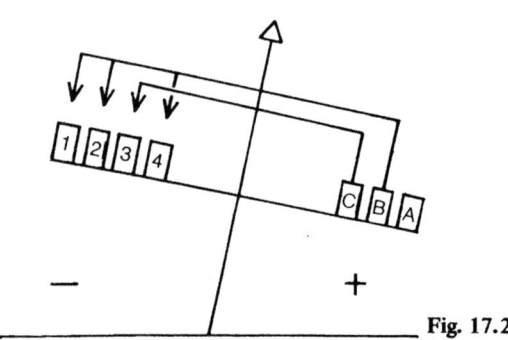

Fig. 17.2

Anaesthesia and operating rooms should be peaceful places where the patient can feel that doctors and nurses are in full control of the situation. Noise and confusion will ruin any effort to prepare the patient positively for anaesthesia. If possible, the patient should be brought to regard anaesthesia and the operation as positive procedures for his getting better. Pre-anaesthetic psychological care and positive influence on the part of doctors and nurses will help the anaesthetist to produce sound and relaxed sleep.

His central nervous system will be relaxed, he will require less anaesthesia, recover faster and get up sooner, which is desired as much by the hospital staff as by the patient.

It is not only easier to anaesthetise a positively prepared patient, but it is necessary to achieve by patient persuasion a challenge to the general attitude of the community towards anaesthesia and surgery which would make for better social health care in this country.

If the attitude towards hospitals had been better, many lives could have been saved. It is the duty of the anaesthetist and of the doctors and nurses to help to change this attitude: not only by providing medicine to remove a patient's pain, but by striving to influence him positively and convince him of the advantages and necessity of hospitals and operations including anaesthesia. We must help him to overcome his fears, his worries and doubts concerning anaesthesia and surgery; if he has confidence in you, he might eventually forget his maladies and his medicines, but he will never forget you.

References

King M (ed) A symposium from Makererere. Medical care in developing countries. Oxford University Press, London, chap 22:8

Vaughan AB (1969) Anaesthetics. Oxford University Press, Oxford

Eichler J, Kompendium der Anaesthesiologie, Fischer, Stuttgart

Pflüger H (1971) Anaesthesie in der Praxis. Schattauer, Stuttgart New York, pp 17-20

Barth L, Meyer M (1965) Moderne Narkose. Fischer, Stuttgart

Stöcker L (1967) Narkose. Thieme, Stuttgart

Benzer H, Frey R, Hügin W, Mayrhofer O (eds) (1977) Lehrbuch der Anaesthesiologie, Reanimation und Intensivpflege. Springer, Berlin Heidelberg New York

Wieners K, Kern E, Günther M, Burchardi H (1969) Postoperative Frühkomplicationen. Thieme, Stuttgart

Farman JV, Anaesthesia and the E.M.O. System. The English Universities Press

Parkhouse J, Simpson BR (1959) A restatement of anaesthetic principles. Br J Anaesth 31

Boyan CP (1963) General Anaesthesia with minimal equipment. NY State J Med 6

Nolte H et al. (1971) Kenntnisse und Aufgaben der Krankenschwestern und Pfleger in der modernen Anaesthesie. Arbeitstagung in Minden 1971. Thieme, Stuttgart

Infusionstherapie (1974) Leitfaden für Medizinische Assistenzberufe. Boehringer, Mannheim

Erikson E (1969) Illustrated handbook in local anaesthesia. Lloyd Luke Medical Books, London

Gorgaß B, Ahnefeld FW (1980) Der Rettungssanitäter, Springer, Berlin Heidelberg New York

Frey R (1966) Suggestion und Narkose. Psychother Psychosom 14:454-458

Acute Care

Based on the Proceedings of the Sixth International Symposium
on Critical Care Medicine
Editors: B. M. Tavares, R. Frey
1979. 133 figures, 97 tables. XVI, 345 pages
(Anaesthesiology and Intensive Care Medicine, Volume 116)
ISBN 3-540-09210-2

G. M. Bedbrook

The Care and Management of Spinal Cord Injuries

Foreword by R. W. Jackson
With a chapter "Paraplegia in Developing Countries"
1981. 147 figures. XVI, 351 pages
ISBN 3-540-90494-8

C. Burri, F. W. Ahnefeld

The Caval Catheter

With the collaboration of numerous experts
Translated from the German Edition "C. Burri, F. W. Ahnefeld,
Cava Katheter"
1978. 54 figures, 18 tables. VII, 84 pages
ISBN 3-540-08566-1

Clinical Management of Mother and Newborn

Editor: G. F. Marx
1979. 30 figures, 44 tables. XIV, 274 pages
ISBN 3-540-90373-9

Critical Care Medicine Manual

Editors: M. H. Weil, P. L. DaLuz
1978. 73 figures, 48 tables. XXIV, 371 pages
ISBN 3-540-90270-8

Endocrinology in Anaesthesia and Surgery

Editors: H. Stoeckel, T. Oyama
With the Co-operation of G. Hack
1980. 101 figures, 45 tables. XI, 203 pages
(Anaesthesiology and Intensive Care Medicine, Volume 132)
ISBN 3-540-10211-6

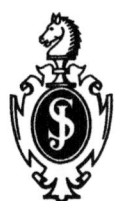

Springer-Verlag
Berlin
Heidelberg
New York

Enzymes in Anesthesiology

Editor: F. F. Foldes
With contributions by numerous experts
1978. 34 figures, 18 tables. XIX, 368 pages
ISBN 3-540-90241-4

D. A. B. Hopkin

Hazards and Errors in Anaesthesia

1980. 5 figures, 2 tables. X, 296 pages
ISBN 3-540-10158-6

F. L. Jenkner

Peripheral Nerve Block

Pharmacologic – By Local Anesthesia. Electric – By Transdermal
Stimulation
Revised and Enlarged Translation of the 2nd German Edition
1977. 72 figures. VII, 116 pages
ISBN 3-211-81426-4

W. S. McDougal, C. L. Slade, B. A. Pruitt, Jr.

Manual of Burns

Medical Illustrators: M. Williams, C. H. Boyter, D. P. Russell
1978. 214 coloured figures, 4 tables. X, 165 pages
(Comprehensive Manuals of Surgical Specialties)
ISBN 3-540-90319-4

Parenteral Nutrition

Editors: F. W. Ahnefeld, C. Burri, W. Dick, M. Halmágyi
Translated from the German by A. Babad
With numerous experts
1976. 103 figures, 64 tables. VIII, 201 pages
ISBN 3-540-07518-6

L. Wille, M. Obladen

Neonatal Intensive Care

Principles and Guidelines
With a Section on Neonatal Cardiology by H. E. Ulmer
Foreword by A. Merritt
Translated from the German by T. C. Telger
1981. 49 figures, 76 tables. XX, 283 pages
ISBN 3-540-10462-3

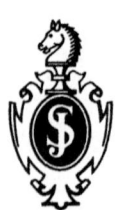

Springer-Verlag
Berlin
Heidelberg
New York